LAWFULLY
ADDICTED

LAWFULLY ADDICTED

CHAIN PHARMACY'S
ROLE IN
OUR OPIOID EPIDEMIC

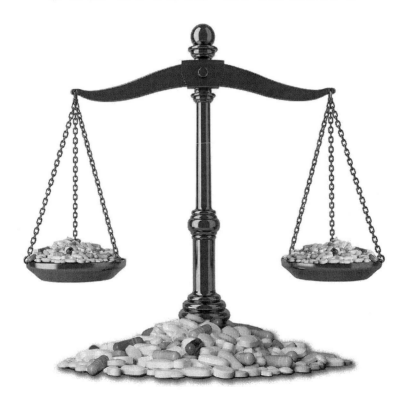

RAYMOND R. CARLSON, R.Ph.

For information about this title or to order other books and/or electronic media, contact the publisher:

Ray Carlson
RayCarlson333@gmail.com

ISBNs:
979-8-9870224-2-9 (hardcover)
979-8-9870224-0-5 (softcover)
979-8-9870224-1-2 (eBook)

Printed in the United States of America

Interior design: 1106 Design
Cover design: Susan Olinsky Design
Edited: Elisabeth Chretien, New York Book Editors

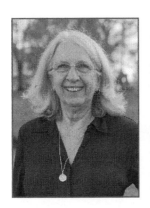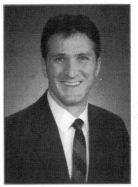

This book is dedicated in memory of my mother, Irene L. Carlson, RN, and my brother Keith L. Carlson, R.Ph.

With Sincere Appreciation to My Wife:
Lori A. Carlson, MS Math
For all her love and support

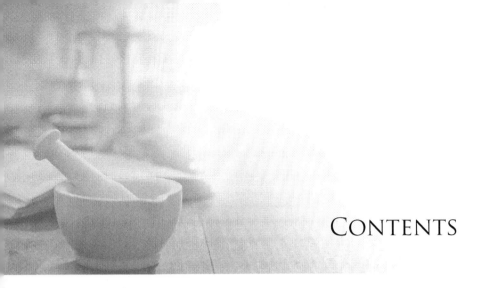

CONTENTS

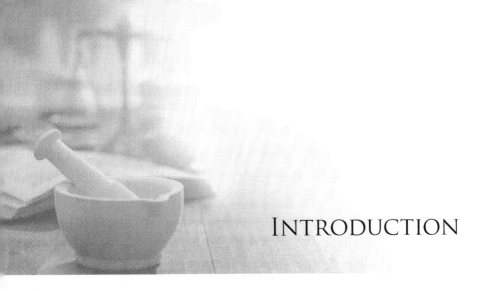

INTRODUCTION

IT'S A FUNNY TWIST OF FATE that men tend to become more feminine as they age and women, more masculine. It's a flip-flopping of testosterone and estrogen that gives each of us a mental and physical taste of the other during our final years. Having recently turned sixty, I hope that my estrogen-filled words can accomplish what my testosterone ones failed to do. During my forty-year career as a pharmacist—and long before the nation's opioid epidemic—I repeatedly warned my colleagues of the consequences of recklessly dispensing prescription drugs without regard for professional standards. I struggle with the thought that I could have helped prevent the resulting crisis if I had sounded the alarm louder.

Our nation's opioid epidemic was not an act of God. It was not nature's way of thinning the herd. It was certainly not because we didn't have laws in place to prevent such a thing from happening. While I cannot speak to the laws that govern other professions, I understand pharmacy law well enough to believe that our nation's misuse of all prescription drugs, including opioids, is aided by chain and employee pharmacists who are skirting the law. I believed this with enough conviction to file a lawsuit against my policing agency, the Ohio Board of Pharmacy (BOP), in 2018. It was as loud an alarm as a pharmacist could sound.

Many are unaware that Congress passed a law in 1990 called OBRA-90, requiring what's known as a "Drug Use Review" (DUR). This law was intended "to thwart the abuse and misuse of prescription drugs." Because corporate pharmacy, driven by the desire to increase profits by any means necessary, ignored the true purpose of this law, pharmacists continued to dispense prescription drugs to patients who should not have received them.

While we are all aware of the "pill mills" that operated in the state of Florida and elsewhere, tens of thousands of licensed pharmacies flying under the radar are operating in a way that is every bit as profit-driven as those pain clinics whose drug-seeking patients formed lines that stretched around street corners in broad daylight. The law clearly states what a licensed pharmacist is supposed to do before handing a prescription drug to a citizen, and while it might be easy for law enforcement to break down the doors of pill mills for the obviousness of their activity, corporate pharmacy's deceit offers the public anything but red-handed violations. Moral hazard violations are difficult to catch, and perpetrators escape accountability because victims trust that the rules of the game are being followed.

The public needs to understand that pharmacy as a profession has drifted away from lawful conduct because the employers most pharmacists work for have made adherence all but impossible. This situation is the perfect example of what we tend to complain about in modern America: degrading jobs, drug abuse, complex corporate structures making billions of dollars, the loss of mom-and-pop shops, healthcare without a human touch, and deception that is hidden in the fine print. Large chain pharmacies have callously abused what used to be our nation's most trusted profession, and in doing so, they have turned corner drug stores into what a court in northeastern Ohio deemed a "public nuisance."

Friends, family, and entire communities have been hit by a tsunami of opioids, and my profession, at its core, is a dispenser of dangerous drugs. In 2021, the United States surpassed 100,000 overdose deaths for the first time in a calendar year. As the public increasingly relies on Google to lessen their ignorance of the medications they take, their need to understand the rules of this profession has never been greater. Corporate pharmacy expects silence from slave-like pharmacists who dispense drugs at a dizzying pace and from ignorant patients who are unable to contrast their pharmacy experience against what the law requires.

My attempts to explain these pharmacy rules to the public on television and radio, on college campuses, and in a lawsuit filed against the Board of Pharmacy all fell on deaf ears, so my hurried pace to fill media time slots has now become these deliberate keystrokes. My journey has given me a unique insight into pharmacy law, the behavior of well-paid and apathetic pharmacists being manipulated by corporate employers, and pharmacy stakeholders who maintain a code of silence. The years I spent fighting my profession's denial of an apparently simple law eventually came to an end when a jury of my peers living in two counties to the north of my hometown offered $650 million worth of vindication to the people in a lawsuit against chain pharmacies.

It is not my intention to make unsubstantiated claims of deceit. I offer plenty of evidence and testimony to back up my claims. Besides, since seventy percent of you take at least one prescription drug per month, read the rules yourself and pay attention in a week or two when you have your next prescription filled, then decide for yourself.

With seventy-five percent of opioid addictions having begun with prescription drugs, and laws put in place decades ago that were supposed to prevent drug abuse, contrast your monthly trip to the pharmacy with this new-found knowledge and look for a connection.

Corporate chain pharmacies can deceive the public because the public does not know about these laws. Should, however, the public take the time to understand the manner in which pills are supposed to be placed in a bottle, and if corporate pharmacy underestimates the extent to which the people have enlightened themselves, they will be sued for the wrong pills their hurried pharmacists dispense, the drug reactions that patients experience without first being warned, or their child who has become addicted. By sharing my personal pharmacy journey and the barriers I ran into along the way, the burden of change might finally land where it belongs: in the hands of people who have a judicial club in their grasp and are ready to swing it.

Now, in the settling dust of "I told you so," and despite the ever-increasing death rates from prescription drug overdoses and drug misuse, I can write about this journey that began with and was shaped by pressing my typewriter keys in a fraternity in 1982. The war of words I waged against self-indulgence while in college continued for decades as I moved from one pharmacy job to another, battling pharmacists who seemed opposed to speaking up about what was going on around them.

◆ ◆ ◆

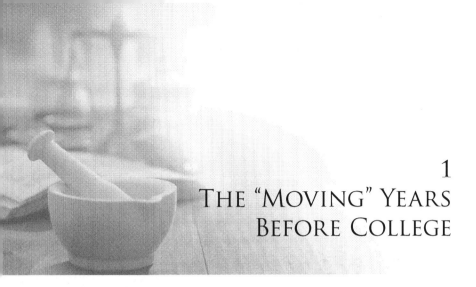

1
THE "MOVING" YEARS
BEFORE COLLEGE

GROWING UP, I WAS NOT WHAT MANY REFER TO as an "alpha
male." I was neither mentally astute enough to nor physically able
to lead the pack. Whether you chalk it up to the junior high show-
ers of the '70s that scarred those of us who were late to develop,
complex hormonal differences that determine rates of maturity,
or my mother's nurturing, I was the small, skinny one who followed behind the group on the sidewalk, trying to insert my humor
into theirs. Although I thought myself somewhat funny, without
the ability to either physically protect the pack or make good on
conversations involving procreation, my place was in the rear
of the group.

My family's home in Kingsville, Ohio, in the early 1970s was
dubbed the "Big House." I suppose all childhood homes seem larger
than they really are, but this house was large enough to easily accommodate my parents and us six children. Just like the Brady Bunch, we
were the "Carlson Kids," three boys and three girls all born within
five years. I was the fifth born. We lived near Lake Erie in northeast
Ohio, playing outside until dark and enjoying our youth. At age ten,

I didn't understand the Vietnam War, going off the gold standard, or climbing interest rates.

My move from Kingsville Elementary School to Braden Junior High in 1974 did not help lay a foundation of self-confidence. Although I don't remember it, we must have taken some kind of aptitude test prior to transitioning to junior high, and I must not have scored well. I was not placed in Section AA or BB, even A or B, but L for "Last." I didn't pay much attention to the designation, though. I thought myself to be a normal twelve-year-old boy, even though my first "ear tag" had indicated that I was different.

Things began to change prior to my beginning eighth grade. That's when our family moved from the Big House into a small two-bedroom apartment several miles away. It was difficult leaving our neighborhood friends and the small town of Kingsville that we had come to love. With much of our furniture stored in my grandmother's basement, my parents somehow managed to cram all eight of us into a four-hundred-square-foot apartment. We lived on the second floor and had a balcony from which we could watch the other children in the complex play outside. I'm not sure why my parents wouldn't let us play outside at first, but the cage-like environment must have worn on us all because they eventually lifted the ban.

Nothing was right about that time in our lives. The bus rides to and from school highlighted the differences between houses and apartments, rich and poor, and I was beginning to understand my place in the world. The tuna-noodle casseroles we often ate for dinner were a testament to the financial difficulties of raising six children. The eighth grade is about when poor kids start to recognize that they're poor. I was starting to put two and two together. Knowing that my bus ride was taking me from a tiny apartment to a classroom labeled "L" had unescapable consequences. It was a mix of poverty and the assumed ignorance shown to me by junior high academia that I would one day have to shrug off. It's the sort of stuff that determines one's ability to make eye contact during conversations or a presentation in front of a class.

Still, I found myself able to forge friendships and participate successfully in extracurricular activities. I was the small, coordinated one who did backflips on the trampoline, could spin a basketball on my finger, and climb the rope to the gym ceiling without the use of my legs. My happy place was the gymnasium because I was coordinated and showing off my dexterity gave me what I needed to balance out other aspects of my life.

Our cramped conditions in the apartment lasted only until my parents found a home we could rent. Once that happened, we moved a few miles closer to my junior high. Once again, I had to begin the befriending ritual in a new neighborhood. My siblings and I didn't care, though. We were out of the tiny apartment and in a small three-bedroom house. The neighborhood was welcoming, and soon enough, I was spending the night at friends' houses.

The summer of 1976 was my favorite. I was heading into ninth grade at Braden Junior High, had a sense of normalcy at home, and was making new friends in a neighborhood that I would have been content to live in for the remainder of my school days. Still the person following behind the pack on the sidewalk, I was at least part of the most respected pack and felt protected in their midst.

That year, I would forge bonds that remain to this day, but this experience was short-lived. My father was a salesman for a paint and wallpaper store ninety minutes away in Youngstown, Ohio, and he was making that drive six days a week from our home in Ashtabula. We saw very little of him during those years. He always had a company car to drive—one of those compact Japanese vehicles that was upsetting the U.S. auto industry at the time—and it always seemed to have a gutter roof rack welded to its frame. The winter of 1976–77 was one of the coldest on record in Ohio, and Route 11, which linked Ashtabula and Youngstown, was a desolate stretch of nothingness. Considering the flimsy company car my father drove, my parents were likely worried about his safety when they made the decision to move us closer to where he worked. It was our third move in four years, but this time, my siblings and I were in high school and well established. Unfortunately, this move meant that I was leaving all my friends to start over again in a town where I knew no one.

I would have protested the move if I'd understood what it meant to attend a new school in a town an hour away. Probably relishing the drama of it all, I was a big help to my parents with my willingness to help pack boxes. My older sisters, who were beginning their junior and senior years, were not so accommodating. Theirs was one for the emotional record books, and they made no bones about refusing to go. Their tantrums and arguments with my parents were understandable, and if they could sneak a ride back to Ashtabula, they were gone. As for me, I shook my friends' hands, climbed into the truck, and off to Canfield I went with a clean slate. There would be no academic expectations of Section L.

My father was a great salesman. He could "sell ice to an Eskimo," as a popular saying at the time went, though we sometimes wondered why he couldn't sell to Eskimos who lived a little closer to the friends we had left behind.

At the time of our move, my mother had just graduated from Kent State's nursing program, and she immediately found a job at Northside Hospital in Youngstown. We were living in the poor section of this wealthy suburb, but now, we at least had my mother's income to help move us along. We were in the midst of a major recession, with 10 percent interest rates on home loans, and gasoline was being rationed according to the license plate numbers. So, as difficult as it must have been for my parents to move us to an area where we knew no one, there were sound economic reasons behind it, and looking back, it may have been the best thing for me. Certainly, it determined my future path.

Youngstown, Ohio, was known for making steel. The huge factory complexes began on the Mahoning River at the Ohio/Pennsylvania state line in a small Ohio town called Lowellville and continued upriver for several miles through Campbell, Struthers, and Youngstown. The water was so polluted that no animals lived in it and no plants could grow around it. Homes within a mile of its banks were painted with the soot that poured from the factory smokestacks. Many tolerated the filth and referred to the air as "smelling of money." Unfortunately, this area of northeastern Ohio was about to become part of our nation's "Rust Belt," and our move to Youngstown that summer coincided with the beginning of the end for steel manufacturing in the Mahoning Valley.

"Black Monday" occurred in Youngstown, Ohio, the morning of September 19, 1977, one month into my sophomore year at my new school in Canfield. The sudden closing of the Campbell Works left five thousand steel mill employees looking for work overnight. Other portions of other mills along the river would also close in the coming weeks, as would all the feeder businesses that relied on them, leaving thousands more unemployed. There was no concept of "too big to fail" back then, and the closing of a business was seen as a natural economic process to shed the inefficient—a necessary evil of sorts. The Youngstown area already had a reputation for being a tough mafia town, and it was about to become even tougher. For us Carlsons, we had just moved into an area that was now reeling from the closure of a major employer, and many of the unemployed were the parents of students attending Canfield High.

The Youngstown community vocally expressed its frustration over what it saw as an unnecessary closure, and labor groups and the employees themselves made several attempts to reopen the mills. When those attempts failed, anger made headlines in the local newspaper. The unemployed took turns with a sledgehammer, smashing the same type of imported Japanese compact car that my father drove. It was a public display of unity amid despair and a clever way to show the community how buying cheap imports negatively affected the working class.

My three years at Canfield High were not without friends, though when I look back, I realize that this period of my life was when I had a great deal of alone time with my projects. I acclimated to my new surroundings as best I could, but I was immature and underdeveloped for my age and still had not found academics to be of much use. I enjoyed playing baseball for Canfield, was cut from their basketball team in the final round and had long-since lost the desire to play football because of a nasty hit I had taken while returning a punt my freshman year. My frame of mind to deliver brutality matched my skeletal frame, which seemed not to want to receive it either. I attended only a handful of basketball and football games during those three years. We each have our own comfort level with crowds, and mine was low at the time.

My best friend, another Ray, helped me find a summer job at an aging amusement park called Idora Park in 1978. I was the ride operator for the bumper cars, and after a couple of years, I worked my way up to relieving other ride operators so they could take their scheduled breaks.

The park's famous Wildcat roller coaster was a heart-throbbing old wooden coaster that I rode probably a thousand times. One day, I thought I could safely experience the ride while sitting on the back of the seat, rather than in it. Predictably, I lost my grip during the fast horseshoe turn and pulled myself back into the seat at the last possible moment before being thrown eighty feet to the ground below. At the time, I had just turned eighteen and was beginning to act according to hormonal secretions that would not peak until I reached my sophomore year in college.

It was during my final year of working at Idora Park—and one of the last years this famous park would remain open—that I decided I wanted to be a pharmacist. My older brother Keith had recently failed out of Ohio Northern University's College of Pharmacy, so maybe it was sibling rivalry that helped me make my decision?

Suddenly, it hit me that I had not taken my high school studies seriously and that I was unprepared for such an academically challenging profession. In my pathetic attempt to catch up, I brought chemistry books to work to read while operating the various rides. Whenever the girls who worked in Kidde Land walked past my ride while on their breaks, I would bury my head in a book, hoping to give the impression that I was going to break the bonds of carny life and make something of myself.

During my senior year of high school, my father's boss owned a beautiful mansion in Mill Creek Park, just down the road from Idora Park, that was empty and for sale. A glass sunroom door located at the rear of the house was mistakenly left unlocked just long enough for me and a couple friends to gain entry. We thought it would be the perfect place to host a senior party. Without permission, we planned the party, handed out maps to help classmates find the mansion, and bought kegs of beer to consume when they got there.

Unfortunately, the glass door that was always unlocked was locked the day of the party, and I paused for just a moment before breaking it to gain entry. The whole thing would probably have gone under the radar were it not for the number of classmates who showed up. No one called the cops, but a physician who lived next door to the mansion worked with my mother, and he found the discarded maps with my name and contact information and suggested to my mother that it must have been me. I was busted.

Having to pay to replace the glass window and carpeting didn't upset my father as much as the fact that I had included my contact information on the maps. I never thought to play the father-son masculinity card and tell my dad that at the age of eighteen I was no longer a virgin and had not participated in the destruction . . . except for breaking the glass. The chemistry books had worked, even though I was meeting with a lawyer to make amends.

I graduated from Canfield High School in 1980 without a single member of my family in the audience, and after having won an award for hosting the best senior class party. Ironically, I would head off to college as someone who wasn't really interested in partying. I'd attended only the senior party I threw, and I didn't exactly participate in it. I was in the quiet company of a female for the very first time while others were downstairs putting their cigarettes out in the beautiful cream-colored carpeting.

After a summer of cold shoulders from my parents, I was leaving for college with a sour taste in my mouth for drunk and disorderly conduct. Although I should have learned my lesson about breaking and entering, later in life, I would repeat the same mistake and break a glass window to enter a place I should not have been in. With my hormones raging in the summer of 1980, I was rambunctious, yet tempered by a mistake, and on my way to the prestigious Ohio Northern University's Raabe College of Pharmacy.

◆ ◆ ◆

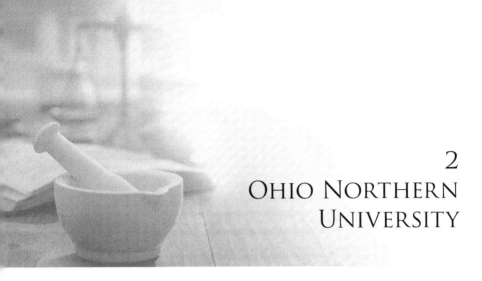

2
OHIO NORTHERN UNIVERSITY

My PARENTS OFTEN SAID that we were unable to visit family because six children were a lot to handle and it was difficult to fit eight bodies into a car. Due to our family's solitude, I never got to know the man I was named after, my great-uncle Raymond Robert Carlson, R.Ph., on my father's side. He graduated from Ohio Northern University's College of Pharmacy in 1941 and joined the U.S. Navy as a pharmacist's mate shortly after Pearl Harbor. He walked ashore at Nagasaki as part of an expeditionary force after the second atomic bomb was dropped. He would describe the experience as "walking on the moon," and that was about all he would say about it. He was still working in a drug store in Ashtabula at the time I applied to pharmacy school, and up until then, I had met him only a few times.

My grades and SAT scores were average, and neither were probably enough to get me into ONU were it not for Uncle Ray's name on a plaque outside the dean's office in recognition of money he had donated. My older brother Keith had lasted only one year at ONU. Now, it was my turn to avoid his fate. I was confident I could learn, even though my GPA didn't always reflect that, and since a pharmacy education required the variety of classes that were of interest to me, I hoped for the best. I was packing up my stuff to move once again, but this time, I was entering a dorm at Ohio Northern University to begin my studies.

I went off to college having been drunk only once on New Year's in 1980, and without having shared an alcoholic drink with my parents. I was unprepared for a college culture that seemed to immerse itself in alcoholic beverages. I didn't know that 0.08 blood alcohol is the point at which the thinner nerves that are responsible for maintaining socially appropriate behavior become impaired and that as levels climb higher, the thicker nerves responsible for maintaining speech and balance are also affected. I was caught off guard by what was probably a blood alcohol level of 0.2 when I lost my balance in the bathroom and knocked out a window on the third floor of Founder's Hall my freshman year.

I blamed this ignorance of alcohol on my parents' decision to pull me away from my junior high friends. My time in high school was spent making new friends and not learning my boundaries in the comfort of old ones. It's that special bond between kindergartners who pee their pants together that allow the walls of embarrassment to fall during times of experimentation years later. Without the closeness of high school friends and the peer pressures that drive new discoveries and with no moments of tipsiness with my parents, I was self-taught in the field of alcohol, and I found that I didn't like it much.

The bags I brought to ONU's Founder Hall were barely unpacked when a friend of my brother Keith knocked on the door of my dorm room. It was Steve Salo from my hometown of Kingsville. I knew him and was glad to see a familiar face. He was a member of the Kappa Psi fraternity, and they were on the hunt to recruit new members for their fraternity. The ritual of "pledging" a fraternity had begun for me, and I entered the trial period in which they wined and dined me before deciding if I was a good fit for their group. I received three invitations to pledge various fraternities, but I chose Kappa Psi because it was a professional pharmacy fraternity and not just a social organization.

Keith lasted only one year at ONU because he overindulged in socializing and partying; unfortunately, neither he nor my parents warned me against this path. No one told me there would be a swarm of fraternity brothers seeking out pledges at all hours, or I would have been prepared for the knocks at the door. Even if I had been warned, I was in a new environment and wanted gang protection as much as fraternities wanted new members. It was difficult for me to resist what I'm certain was responsible for the failure of many who, like my brother, were more interested in partaking in social rituals than studying for exams.

After witnessing the activities of their children, most parents would agree that the prefrontal cortex of the brain does not mature until around age twenty-five. A female's high estrogen levels compared with a male's can speed this process up a bit, but for the most part, it's at age twenty-five. The prefrontal cortex is what adults use to think rationally and override other, more emotionally or instinctually driven areas of the brain, such as the amygdala. The prefrontal cortex develops based on past experiences, and eventually, we have enough accumulated memories of good and bad experiences and outcomes to guide us into doing what isn't always easiest.

We are all lucky to survive the delayed development of our prefrontal cortex while the rest of our reptilian brain is bathed in adolescent hormone juices, and while I was not thinking this exact thought at my first fraternity party, I was feeling uncomfortable with the activity I was seeing for the first time. I saw the same mob-like activity at the frat party that I had seen in the mansion owned by my father's boss, and my tinge of Asperger's just knew that it wasn't for me. I was eighteen years old and could not explain why I was feeling this way, and yet at age forty I wished I would have fought those feelings more and relaxed enough to enjoy that time of my life. But I didn't, and I continued down the path of fraternity life despite my early inclinations to do otherwise.

The ritual of pledging had begun, and by the winter of 1981, I was jogging around campus singing songs, cleaning the Kappa Psi fraternity house, and serving as an alarm clock at ungodly hours, only to have profanities shouted at me to come back in ten minutes. I was the upperclassmen's snooze button in a crude sort of way, but it was just one of the many tests they dished out to pledges to see if we would weaken and quit.

Not every brother in the fraternity was this way. Some were very kind, but you could tell those who had it in them to be the nasty type. Maybe the brothers divided themselves into "nasty" or "nice" roles by a show of hands prior to rush? Either way, it was a play that lasted for ten weeks and involved several scenes that were scripted to move one from feelings of brotherly love to those of anger and division. The sole purpose was to demonstrate that division could never exist within the brotherhood.

"Hell week" began prior to the beginning of the spring semester, and us pledges had to return to ONU early for "boot camp." During Hell Week, I found myself sleeping for only a few hours at a time on the floor of the laundry room. With all the "yes sirs" and "no sirs" I addressed to drill sergeant-like brothers, and the pushups I had to do for bad behavior, it was obvious to me that this ritual was developed by brothers who had served in the military years ago. It was the ultimate "Us vs. Them" dynamic, staged at the expense of the pledges, and with the purpose of creating a band of brothers. The division had climaxed on the final day with a fight between those brothers we thought to be protecting us and those who wanted to punish us, and with punches thrown and a window broken, myself and the two other pledges with me were swept away to a safe house for protection.

We all collapsed from exhaustion on the floor of Steve's house. Awoken from a dead sleep, we were taken back to the KY frat house one at a time, led into a candle-lit room, ordered to sit in front of gothic-looking features, and questioned about our devotion. Tears burst from my eyes when I was informed that this was all a play and that I was now a brother. Nothing but hugs and handshakes remained for me that evening, and few events in my life were as happy and as seemingly significant as that one. Hell week had ended, and I was now a brother.

I was now very behind in my studies and distanced myself shortly after Hell week in an effort to catch up. Knowing that my parents wouldn't let me return if I teetered on the edge of passing, I buried my head in books instead of running around softball fields and attending fraternity meetings. On Mother's Day 1981, I wrote my mother a letter, telling her that I loved her, that I was doing my best to make her proud of me, and that I had managed to bring my grades up at the expense of receiving notice from the KY brotherhood that they were going to vote on whether to kick me out for not attending their functions. I survived the vote, attended their meetings, and paid a price, like my brother Keith had.

My spring quarter at ONU did not go as well as my parents wanted it to. Although I managed to obtain the minimum 2.00 GPA that was required to continue in the pharmacy college, it was not enough to satisfy my parents, who struggled to pay for my tuition. The 'D' I received in calculus—although numerically balanced by my

'B' in Biology—was not going to cut it. I had succumbed to the same fate as my brother and would not be returning to ONU in the fall. I blamed myself and the fraternity for it.

I was not a prepared student, and I could not afford anything but total dedication to my studies. The time I had wasted in high school meant that I should have dedicated all my time to learning while in college. I should have been visiting professors' offices and asking questions instead of cleaning a fraternity. I should have been waking myself up for class instead of waking a fraternity brother whose only fraternal purpose was to make me feel bad about myself and have me do pushups if I was late or early or loud or silent. I don't know what I was thinking, but obviously, I was not thinking about the pharmacy curricula. I would have to prove myself the following year at Youngstown State University if I ever hoped to see the sidewalks of ONU again and perhaps one day work behind a pharmacy counter.

I attended YSU for my second year of college and did well enough for my parents to give me a second chance. If I did well while attending a summer session at ONU, they would allow me to stay for the fall semester. The class I took at ONU the summer of 1982 was anatomy/physiology with Dr. Reggie McGraw, and he was known for being tough—extremely tough. I lived at the fraternity that summer and existed on ramen noodles and Chef Boyardee pasta. I was taking one of the university's toughest year-long classes, taught by one of ONU's most challenging professors, crammed into a single summer, and I would handle it like a pro.

I ate, drank, and slept human anatomy that summer and exceeded 100 percent on two of the three crammed sessions. I taped each lecture with my small cassette recorder and hurried back to the fraternity after class each day to mark up my notes with different colored pens. I loved every bit of information I received, and I felt as though there was little Dr. McGraw could ask that I could not answer. I had never experienced education like this before; nothing was memorized and regurgitated. We learned in a way that made me appreciate for the first time why I was attending college. It was the academic awakening that had escaped me in high school, and this class and its subject matter were important enough to support me through many of the classes I had yet to take. I had learned how the human body worked, and from then on, I would be able to compete in the classroom.

I had the pleasure of spending that quiet summer of '82 at the KY house, absent the rest of the brotherhood, with the brilliant companionship of brother Peter Wong. It was the first time I had lived in the frat house, and I knew that the fraternal environment the few of us in the house enjoyed that summer wouldn't last long once the rest of the brotherhood returned. I was ready this time, however, since I felt myself to be on a similar academic plane as the others. Most were valedictorians of their high schools and probably didn't have to study as much as I did. But now, I knew what I had to do to make it, and if my parents were willing to continue paying my tuition, I wasn't going to let them down. More importantly, I wasn't going to let myself down by underestimating the amount of study time I needed amidst the fraternal distractions of brotherhood. If I had any spare time, I planned to dedicate it to other pharmacy-related activities more suitable to my interests. I was still a brother and the frat house was my home, for better or worse.

I had my college epiphany because I was away from the influences of the fraternity, which, in my mind, played a role in my returning home for my second year. While I was away, I didn't receive a single phone call from any of my "life-long brothers," so it was easy for me to have a change of attitude toward the meaning of brotherhood. I began to distance myself from brotherly interactions and focused instead on my studies. I saw the fraternity as a distraction getting in the way of my goal, and I did an about-face.

I recognized that there was too much play in my fraternal environment and not enough work. It was a constant competition to see who was the funniest, and I was rarely in the mood to entertain the endless barrage of jokes. If I could have moved the fraternal masses to organize a charity event as readily as they threw a toga party, I could have tolerated the "work hard, play hard" justification. Studying was hard work and pharmacy was a challenging curriculum, but I was not seeing the balance, or at least not one that suited my academic abilities.

"Fraternity Circle" at ONU was lined with frat houses at the time, and several others were scattered throughout campus side streets. The partying was not limited to the fraternities and those who joined them. There was an unmistakable campus culture of self-indulgence, and although a small part of me regrets not having relaxed enough to soak some of that pleasure in, I didn't. For whatever reason, I simply couldn't. Maybe I was not afforded the luxury of play because of my Section L past? And if others were either genetically gifted or had already put in their academic time in high school, I often wondered how much higher they could have climbed. Many would not climb at all, and nearly two thirds of my pharmacy class would change majors or disappear from campus altogether.

Perhaps my resistance to giving in to all this hedonism was due in part to all the plant closings back home or the financial struggles my parents had in raising six children. Our country had started losing good manufacturing jobs and replacing them with retail shops, bars, and restaurants. We were entering a golden age of consumption, and the loss of good manufacturing jobs turned workers who once made steel shelves into workers who stocked them. In this context, the desire to party and play felt like an omen of bad things to come.

Our fraternity, like many others at that time, was taking binge drinking to new heights, and although I participated on occasion, most of my memories of parties are of standing along the wall by myself, thinking about how college campuses had once been the place where social change ignited. Thoughts of the movie *Animal House* would change my mood in an instant, and since no one likes having a stick in the mud hanging around a party, I would soon leave.

There was no reason in the early '80s for any of us to think that dark times were ahead. Pharmacy jobs were abundant, and salaries were some of the highest available right out of school. Once we had our sheet of paper from the university, and our license from the Board of Pharmacy, we could throw a dart at a map and know we could begin our lives there as a pharmacist. Although it is different today, back then we experienced very little while working our summer pharmacy intern jobs to cause us to have second thoughts about our chosen profession, and academia had no murky future to gloss over when questioned about what we students were seeing in the real world. All seemed rosy for pharmacy students, and most had every reason to enjoy what lay ahead.

Pharmacy students were returning to their parents' pharmacy to work during their holiday and summer breaks and would return to classes intending to one day experience similar levels of prosperity. If a student was interning for a chain pharmacy, their experience was like that of independents. The prescription volumes were reasonably similar, computers and insurance hassles had yet to arrive, and chain pharmacists still had the ability to make professional decisions regarding services and staffing. Back then, students and academia did not question whether the knowledge obtained in the classroom would be used. The profession and it's organizations were dominated by independent pharmacists, and it seemed protected at the time.

I was in my P-3 year in 1982 and working as a pharmacy intern for Revco Drug. The stores I floated to seemed rather small and independent-like. The pharmacists I worked under were all pleasant, showed little signs of stress, and were making lots of money. We were not filling crazy numbers of prescriptions per day because we were still using paper cards to keep track of patient profiles. Without the advent of computers, patient care was a manual task that required time. Without gigabytes of data storage available to a pharmacist, human interaction was a must, and pharmacist's memory of patient conditions, previous drugs taken, adverse reactions, etc. provided the necessary storage. I was happy working for the Revco Drug chain and planned to continue once I graduated.

I had as much reason as others to party when I thought my timing and mood was right, but in my P-3 year I began to immerse myself in student professional organizations, and attended my first American Pharmacists Association (APhA) Annual Meeting in Montreal and my first Ohio Pharmacists Association Annual Meeting in Akron. As a student representative from ONU to both organizations, I was catching wind of problems within pharmacy that caused me concern. And although I may not have understood what pharmacists were arguing about at various house of delegates and board meetings, I knew something was up. Funny as it may seem, it was pharmacists from my hometown, our "Rust Belt," who seemed to be the most vocal during meetings, and their anger established a baseline of concern in my young brain. I would return to ONU after each meeting with a sense of urgency even if I did not truly understand the reasons why.

Binge drinking was not on my mind, only what I thought were motivating words to fellow pharmacy students and the keys on my typewriter that I needed to press to write them. It would be fair to say that at times I was offensive, but I found others to be the same and I felt myself only offensive toward their offenses.

Although I'm giving the impression that I had constant conflict with the KY brotherhood, this was not the case at all. I bonded with most of them in one way or another and I enjoy friendships that remain to this day. I lived in the KY house for a year, made extra money keeping the kitchen clean after meals, and attended as many social events as my time would allow. I meant no offense, nor did they to me, and so doors were left open to friendship. I had an inner struggle that was based on my worries for the future, and as much as I wish I had not been burdened by it, I could not rid myself of it.

In the spring of 1983, my inner turmoil met up with a 2 AM incident while I was sleeping and necessitated my asking the dean of students, Bill Robinson, to allow me to move out of the fraternity and into an off-campus apartment. Yes, I think I have a jovial personality, and no, I never had a steady girlfriend to show to others. And "to each his own" as far as I care, so I never really took offense or was bothered by the late-night advance, but it came at a time when I was ready to say goodbye to fraternity living and do my own thing. Permission to leave was granted and I found a single bedroom apartment overtop a grocery store on Main Street. I was able to focus on what I wanted to accomplish academically and professionally, and although I remained friends with many of the brothers, I was free to run for a leadership position in a student organization.

◆ ◆ ◆

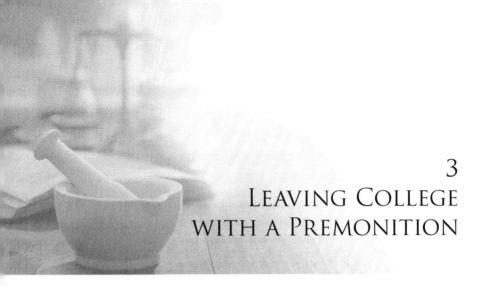

3
LEAVING COLLEGE
WITH A PREMONITION

I HAVE AN OLD PICTURE OF MYSELF at age twenty-one, sitting behind a typewriter at Ohio Northern University, all wound up and trying to stir the emotions of my fellow pharmacy students. That image seems like as good a place as any to begin the professional side of my story. I had found myself on solid academic footing in my third year of college and was involved in student professional associations enough to feel as though I could run for office.

The first student office I sought my P-3 year was that of president of ONU's student branch of the American Pharmacists Association (Student APhA). I remember everyone's heads down on their desks as we raised our hands to vote, and the feeling somewhat surprised to learn that I had won when we raised them. I was elected president of our Student APhA chapter and would take office my following P-4 year. As president, I automatically had a seat on ONU's Student Senate as a representative to the pharmacy college. It was the first step that would lead to miles of activism for the profession of pharmacy, and I would spend the summer thinking about ways to make money for our group and increase professional activity.

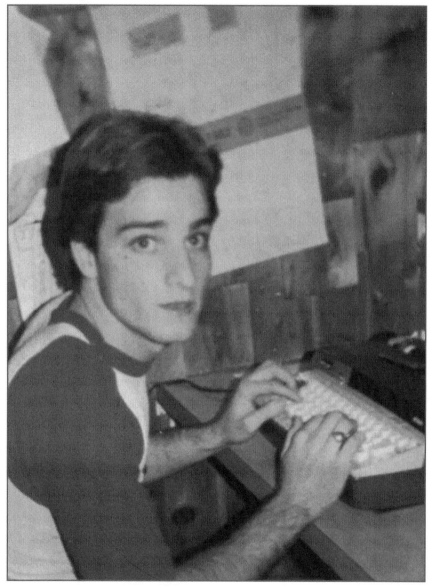

Ray at Kappa Psi Fraternity—1982

When I returned for the fall semester in 1983 as a P-4, professional association activity had me writing bulletins and organizing fundraisers within our college of pharmacy. The keys of my typewriter were busy generating mailings and notices of meetings, along with the poetry I was sending to a sorority girl who lived across the street. It was ONU's homecoming, and time to build our student APhA homecoming float for the parade. I had collected dozens of bags of used prescription vials over the summer while working at Revco Drug as an intern, and I thought I would use them to adorn our float. There were no HIPAA laws back then, but I still had the presence of mind to peel off the prescription labels .

As busy as I was, I didn't notice that the electricity was disconnected in my apartment until my typewriter failed to turn on. When that happened, I ran an extension cord across the hall into a kind neighbor's outlet until Monday morning, when I could pay the bill and have power restored. I could function without electricity, but when my water was shutoff, the days it took to turn it back on seemed an eternity. Man's hierarchy of needs (water) became evident to me, and I was too embarrassed to ask for help from the neighbor next door.

While dozens of our fraternity brothers were busy constructing our float for the homecoming parade, I was one of only three student APhA members who volunteered to help construct our organization's float. It was a long cold night next to a fire with two wasted kegs of beer, that I spent alone trying to get glue to dry on large cardboard panels, to which I had affixed thousands of prescription bottles in patterns. I pulled an all-nighter trying to finish the float. I was cold, wet, and smelled like smoke when I handed the keys to the old Cadillac that formed the basis of our float to another member of our group to drive in the parade. I collapsed on the couch in my second-story apartment overlooking Main Street and awoke only briefly to the sound of the band below before drifting off again. We won third place, and I had slept through it all.

The poor turnout for working on the float was the first nail of professional apathy to be driven into my side. More would come in the years ahead, but this was the first time I would witness an unequal distribution of professional and social time, and I think I was more shocked than hurt. I had worked hard to provide a cool, fun setting in which to build our professional association's float, and almost no one had showed up to help, to converse about issues or not, and to build something other pharmacy students would see and want to involve themselves in. Instead, my professional fraternity brothers, as well as the rest of our student APhA membership, sought the path of least professional resistance.

Nobody likes a critic, yet I was about to play my first role as one. I had further distanced myself from the fraternity that year, and I was about to be called out for it. What began as one of my greatest accomplishments as a young adult—surviving hell week and gaining a brotherhood—soon turned into a source of confrontation and bitter feelings. My life-long status of KY brotherhood was in jeopardy and at risk of being stripped from me.

My verbal criticisms—I never put them in writing—had gotten back to our fraternal leaders, and they decided to put me on trial to have me officially removed from the fraternity. I probably deserved every bit of justice they thought I had coming. I was bitter toward the brotherhood for their poor attendance and participation in pharmacy association meetings, and they were upset with me because I was not attending their fraternity meetings and social events.

During my first year as brother, the brotherhood had voted whether to keep me as a member because I missed more meetings than what our fraternity bylaws allowed. My infraction this time around must have elevated my offense, and now that I was to be dealt with under Section C, Subsection 2b, as a "second offender." Who knows? But a simple vote would be elevated to a trial of sorts with witnesses for both the prosecution and defense. Since I held little inclination to attend and was wishing that I could have stripped away their membership status in Student APhA for not attending meetings and events, those who spoke on my behalf outnumbered those against, and I was allowed to maintain my KY membership status. I was not without the feeling of embarrassment, and yet I knew that no matter the outcome, I would continue to shake the hands of certain brothers in a manner consistent with tradition. I was busy at that time and would not hold it against them.

Again, I might be giving the impression that I was some condescending dweeb who sat in judgment of others, that I couldn't relax and drink an alcoholic beverage because of some demon that haunted me, or that I thought the world was soon coming to an end. I'm a Libertarian at heart, can party with the best when the reasons are right to do so, and I have always had an optimistic view of the world. I have no demons that keep me from seeing the best in people, from enjoying life, or that strip me of hope for the future to such extent that I would not work to make it better.

What I cannot change about my DNA is the quid pro quo attitude I have that focuses on cause and effect. I was expected to be an active member in a fraternity because I had joined it and was expected by that organization to be one. Similarly, those who join a professional association and list membership in it on their resume when they look for a job should be expected to be an active member. I knew the impact my absence would have, and I compared it to the impact their absence had.

I did raise my hand and swear to God to be the best KY member I could be. I repeated a creed that bound me to the expectation that I would attend and participate in the affairs of the brotherhood, and I would promote the fraternal organization and abide by the constitution for which it stood. There was no such swearing in for membership into Student APhA, no swearing to God, and no exchange of blood to bind anyone to active participation. Pharmacy students were free to fill out a form for membership, pay a small membership fee, and left to their own professional conscience to decide if they wanted to show up, run for an office, offer dialog, and better the organization according to the constitution for which it stood. There would be no vote to have them removed, and no trial if they decided never to show their face. Few students would join and participate, and that same conscience would be carried with them after graduation and into their lives as pharmacists.

Is it possible that I was seeing the seeds of our nation's opioid addiction problem planted in college? But who thinks this way at that age, and who could have possibly predicted the number of deaths medication misuse would cause? I was only thinking "tit-for-tat." I was engaged in a simple adolescent argument because I was not going to their meetings and they were not coming to mine. No more and no less back then, and yet it serves as a metaphor today for what would later descend on our profession of pharmacy and the trusting public we would injure.

Pharmacy students decided that planning a hairy buffalo party was more important than planning a fundraiser to help build a stronger community and respectable profession. They chose a "porcelain God" to talk into instead of a microphone. After graduating as a pharmacist and swearing to uphold the laws before boards of pharmacy, they would be absent in even larger numbers from the very organizations that could have protected our communities instead of flushing them.

The year 1984 had arrived and the Orwellian-like state we feared was getting a footing. In just a few years it would be helped along by computers. A future where major industries would be dominated by a few players, large scale corruption, repressive regimentation of activity, and mass surveillance needed only apathy to make it real. Like Y2K in 1999, we talked about what would happen to our computers when the year reached 2000, we spoke of Orwell's 1984 that year while on campus and wondered if it was a possibility. With hindsight being what it is and had my crystal ball been polished enough to offer a glimpse of what things would be like in 2022, I would have attended my fraternity trial and argued my case.

If I had the knowledge of our profession's future in my hand, I would have told them at my trial that over one million lives would be lost to opioid overdose deaths between 1999 and 2022; and their parents' independent pharmacy would close, nearly 10,000 across the U.S. in just six years. I would have warned them that the majority of pharmacy students would be working for chain pharmacies that had cameras behind the counter, phone systems that kept track of how long it took to answer, and their pace of dispensing dangerous drugs would be aided by computer screens that changed color if they took too long to fill a prescription. Their hurried pace, I would warn them of, would see their frustrations about workplace conditions being expressed in the millions on this thing called social media.

How might the brotherhood have felt in 1984 about professional association membership and participation if they knew what their careers would be like in 2022? Would they have thought themselves to be retired by then, and still chose socializing over professional gatherings? Or would they have read what to do in the bylaws of our professional organization and work tirelessly to protect pharmacy the same way they sought to protect the fraternity and remove my presence from it?

If only I (we) had known that after graduation we would eventually be filling one prescription every sixty seconds, and if we had the time to talk to patients, there might be an insurance contract that would forbid us from saying anything negative, there would not have been a trial. They would have attended our meetings, and I would have attended theirs. We would have worked hard together within Student APhA, and we would have played hard together within the fraternity for the accomplishments we would have made. But this is not how it was on campus and not how it would be behind pharmacy counters after graduation.

I'd had my first professional confrontation and narrowly escaped punishment from those who, in my mind, weren't falling in line with this big professional picture I had envisioned. Professional apathy had reared its ugly head in front of me for the first time. The lack of participation and professionalism and even joining for the sake of offering membership support was evident, and it was exchanged for what seemed to be never-ending parties. The brothers tried to laugh off their professional apathy and pretend it didn't exist, only later to hold a trial rich in gothic symbolism to justify their absence from association work based on rituals and tradition. I would remain a brother of the fraternity but would never set foot in the KY house again except to see it a few years after graduation, when it had been forcibly abandoned and left to decay.

A greater good, or at least my idea of a greater good, had taken hold in my mind. Fraternal embarrassment or not, I had discovered the potential benefits of professional association. The constitution and bylaws of the Student APhA were aligned with those that governed this professional pharmacy fraternity, and I wanted to bring the two organizations closer together. After graduation, we were able to join Ohio Pharmacists Association (OPA) and APhA as full-fledged pharmacist members and impact these organizations with all that our elevated status of pharmacists could bring, and yet participation numbers would drop below what was seen on campus. After graduation, I would attend state and national meetings and not be able to tell if there were more pharmacists or students in attendance.

I would spend the next several decades trying to beat down the same kind of professional apathy I saw in the fraternity in a failed attempt to instill confidence and professionalism in those who hold positions of responsibility. This pharmacy student culture would soon "graduate" into a nearly identical pharmacist culture.

I don't know if Kappa Psi ever held a trial to "remove" a "brother" before me. If not, it's not a distinction I'm particularly proud of. Looking back, I probably should have exerted my social skills to address the obviously deteriorating situation before it reached this point. On the other hand, in the end, it may well have helped hone my skills for the professional battles that would follow. In time, Carlson vs. Kappa Psi Fraternity would become Carlson vs. The Ohio State Board of Pharmacy. I moved on from pointing out professional apathy to actively trying to prevent the public harm that resulted from it.

I didn't realize it then, but real challenges were already taking hold of our profession. Even as a student on campus, I saw a serious disconnect between the amount of time pharmacy students spent making our profession better and the time they spent ignoring this necessary effort. It was a noticeable habit that future pharmacists would carry from college campuses to behind pharmacy counters and would eventually result in a professional bondage unlike any other. Most concerning, however, was the level of self-indulgence that blinded these highly educated individuals to the community responsibilities they had pledged themselves to and the pharmacy license to which they were bound. When the public harm caused by the misuse of prescription drugs first presented itself, these professionals were nowhere to be found in the ensuring debate.

Another ONU record I may hold—and this one I am actually proud of—is for pharmacy advocacy, having served on the Student Senate, on the Pharmacy Council, as president of ONU's Student APhA chapter, and as our college representative to the Ohio Pharmacists Association (OPA) Board of Trustees. I had caught the pharmacy bug in a big way and managed to juggle all my responsibilities while still maintaining good grades. Although I graduated in the middle of my class, I was able to absorb enough education to become a clinically versatile pharmacist.

I left campus with a professional association education that money couldn't buy, and more importantly, I understood that education does not end with graduation. Everything I missed in class prior to my educational epiphany would be made up for in spades when my desire to learn on my own kicked in. I would go on to teach myself everything from drug dosing to hormones to pharmacy law, and my appetite for knowledge could not be satisfied, especially when my business or my reputation was on the line. Ohio Northern had given me—and I had taken—all that I could have asked for and more.

Just a few years after my graduation, ONU deactivated its chapter of Kappa Psi Fraternity and turned its house into a maintenance facility for the local park. The unprofessional activity must have continued after I graduated to the point where safety had become a concern for the university. I can now write about the secret rituals of forty years ago because those traditions and rituals are gone.

The premonition I had regarding the fate of our fraternity would eventually be dwarfed by the one I later had for our profession just before the opioid epidemic took hold—only this time, with much more serious consequences. A fraternity closing pales in comparison to a million or more citizen deaths due to overdose, misuse, and abuse of prescription drugs. A generation steeped in self-indulgence would graduate to embrace a culture of apathy, and in doing so, they would create enough public chaos for a court to eventually declare a pharmacy a "public nuisance."

◆ ◆ ◆

4
WELCOME TO THE
PROFESSION OF PHARMACY

My UNCLE RAY WAS A PHARMACIST for Revco Drug and worked in their downtown Ashtabula store for many years. Just as he may have helped me get into ONU, he helped to secure me a job for the same chain he was working for. I was now a graduate pharmacist preparing to take the boards that, when passed, would make me a registered pharmacist (R.Ph.) No amount of college education in pharmacy mattered if you could not pass the boards, so I was studying my anatomy and chemistry books in preparation. I had taken a big leap from operating the bumper cars at Idora Park to putting pills in a bottle while under the supervision of a licensed pharmacist.

Although I recollect a busy pace at the chain pharmacy where I worked—maybe 180 prescriptions a day—it was a much slower pace in 1985 than what I would experience later in my retail pharmacy career. Nothing was automated back then. There were large rolls of labels that fed into a typewriter, and every patient had a customer card in a large filing box, which we used to manually keep track of new and refilled prescriptions. I was an efficient three-fingered typist, so it was easy for me to keep up. There were no computers or printers at the time, almost all customers paid with cash, and the average price for a month's supply of medication was affordable. For the most part, we were able to take the time necessary with each customer to explain the benefits and dangers of the drugs they were about to consume. That dynamic would soon change and change in a big way.

Revco Drug would later become CVS, but at that time, it was still a well-respected company with a good mix of merchandise. Coupons and customer incentives were not overbearing, and prescription insurance companies didn't seem to occupy much of our time processing claims for payment. State Medicaid was easy to process, and we had only a couple of local charity accounts to deal with, which were paid monthly. Company headquarters shouldered much of what we considered to be simple paperwork. Most drugs were covered, pre-authorization was not required, and paper prescription claims went into a blue bag for HQ to deal with. Our only insurance headaches came back to us in little red bags, and we would have to make corrections, mostly clerical in nature, to the prescription claims being billed.

Revco covered a small portion of my tuition while at ONU, and I was obligated to work for them for a certain length of time after graduation in exchange for their cancellation of some of the debt I owed to them. That was not the reason I went to work for them. I enjoyed the company, its leaders, Al Sebok, R.Ph., and Joe Sabino, R.Ph., and the pharmacy staff at the stores I floated to. We were a retail chain establishment with some semblance of a hometown feel, even though the pace was beginning to pick up and supervisors were expecting store managers to call them weekly with new and refill prescription numbers and sales data. If we had a computer, it didn't have the ability to collect and transmit information relating to store performance.

My first indication in 1985 that chain pharmacy was hurting "mom and pop" stores was a phone call I received from an independent pharmacist down the road, wanting to know how and why we were dispensing generic Zantac so cheaply. I felt sorry for the independent pharmacist who was calling to transfer one of his patient's prescriptions to us. We had dozens of bottles of the drug stacked on our shelves because Revco was able to purchase large quantities more cheaply. It seemed to be an unfair advantage and our state pharmacist's association (OPA) would try to tackle by forming a Group Purchasing Organization (GPO) of independent stores. This grouping of independent pharmacies would allow its members to pull their purchasing power to receive the same discounts being offered to the chains, and it would represent one of the first "middlemen" to squeeze themselves between drug suppliers and consumers while taking a slice of the money that was changing hands. Once established, GPOs would take administrative fees and/or collect a percent of all dollars' worth of drugs sold.

These advantages that chain pharmacies had over independents helped begin the race for customer volume. When combined with weekly advertising, coupons, and advertising gimmicks, profitable chain stores soon began filling over two hundred prescriptions with just one pharmacist and a couple techs in a twelve-hour day. While many chain stores continued to fill what many pharmacists would consider reasonable prescription volumes, those that operated closer to urban areas began to push the safe pace of patient dispensing higher. As someone who floated to various stores throughout the county, I could always tell the type of pharmacy operation I was walking into by the bags under the eyes of the pharmacists working there.

When I graduated from ONU in 1985, I was still living in Canfield and working at a Revco Drug nearby in Struthers, Ohio. My mother called me at work one day to let me know that I had received a letter from the Ohio Board of Pharmacy with my exam results. I raced home in the middle of the workday to open it. I had passed the boards and was now a licensed pharmacist (R.Ph.). I yelled with joy, hugged my mom, and headed back to work to deliver the news that I was now able to work behind a pharmacy counter without a licensed pharmacist looking over my shoulder, for I was now licensed myself. Cecelia, the pharmacy manager of the Struthers store, congratulated me and then informed me that she was leaving and that the store would be all mine to manage. She had accepted another pharmacy job and was handing me the keys to go it alone.

There was a big shortage of pharmacists in 1985, and Revco Drug was unable to hire an assistant pharmacist to help cover store hours for the first year I was there. There was simply no one to hire. Pharmacy managers working at other stores were calling every pharmacist they knew to help cover their hours, and it was just a matter of how many hours you wanted to work and how much money you wanted to make that determined whether you took their call. I was young, strong, and full of energy, and I loved the money I was making. My personal record of working thirty-four days straight is one I would never break. I earned around six hundred dollars a week, sixteen hundred in 2022 terms, and loved life with all the extra money I was making. Many of us were enjoying a two-pharmacist income, minus a lot of taxes.

The Revco in Struthers was now my store, and it had a great pace of only about one hundred prescriptions per day. I worked there for a couple of years and was able to build up the business to the point where a busy day topped 150 scripts. I knew my customers' names and histories, and I knew their children well enough to shoot rubber bands at them from behind the pharmacy counter for fun. I received pies around the holidays and cards and gifts on my birthday. There was never an argument between customers and staff. The pace was perfect, and it was a treasured beginning to my pharmacy career.

Struthers is a small town on the Mahoning River just upstream from Lowellville. The entire valley, from Lowellville to Warren, Ohio, was once teaming with facilities that manufactured steel. The buildings were enormous and stretched for miles along the river, with smokestacks that towered over the valley floor. Most of my customers were elderly and retired from those mills, and their stories fascinated me. Many had been employed at the mills on "Black Monday" and sent home abruptly. Tens of thousands of peoples' lives were changed in an instant, and now, all that remained from the decades of steel manufacturing in the area were these huge rusting structures.

My curiosity piqued, I eventually decided that I needed to see these buildings before they were dismantled. I wanted to have a sense of what my customers were talking about.

With testosterone high and this new thing called a camcorder on my shoulder, I would park my jeep on one of the hidden roads leading to the mills and make a dash for the old buildings, past the signs that said "Keep Out." I ran though the graveled fields and over many sets of railroad tracks, climbed my way inside one of the old buildings, and began to film its emptiness. A rush of empathy washed over me, first for those who used to work inside, and then for the sheer size of the structures that were now rusting away. I carefully walked through one arena-sized building after another, my camera rolling the whole time, in absolute awe of what these Americans, my customers, had built. I felt as though I were the size of a flea in a shoe box for the monstrosity of it all, and my heart ached at what I was filming.

The first time I was caught by security, they let me go when I told them who I was and what I was doing. Thinking I had got off pretty lucky, I had to do it again, and this time I would not be so fortunate.

I had recorded myself breaking the glass window through which I reached to unlock the door to the infirmary building. Everything about the place was already ransacked, trashed, and falling apart, and just walking through the debris was at your own peril. But when I saw a healthcare-related building that I had not yet ventured into, I went in. The filing cabinets were full of records, and my camera was recording as I flipped through paperwork, looking for something historically significant. When caught, I offered the same explanation as I had previously, and they let me go after confiscating the tape.

I mention these trespasses because they had a profound impact on me. I empathized with my customers who had been impacted by the closing of so many manufacturing facilities, and I knew the reasons why they had to clip coupons. I saw the blight, the ruined lives, and the change of self-esteem that it surely must have had on those now out of work, and my toolbox was not big enough to make it all better for them. All I could do is try to understand what I was looking at, make the connection between buildings that employed thousands, and remember it when conversing with my patients who might have worked in one.

I still have many of those tapes, and one day, I will go through them and see if there is any historic value to them. At the time, I edited some into music videos (MTV was big at that time) and connected in some small way to my drug-store customers. I also finally learned the lesson that had escaped me in high school when I broke a glass window to enter someone else's property. It was indeed someone else's property, and the owners were wasting no time in cashing in on the money they could make by dismantling the steel buildings and equipment and selling them. A huge company was developed to do just that, and when there was nothing left to dismantle, they went bankrupt.

I was single and had the ability to generate income, and in those days, it was a lot. One day, I drove over to the town immediately east of Struthers, Lowellville, Ohio, which I had never been to before. I noticed that their local pharmacy had just closed its doors. I looked past the broken, boarded-up windows and thought that I could fix it up and open my own mom-and-pop drug store. I had increased sales at the Revco in Struthers, and believing that I enjoyed a great relationship with many customers who lived just a couple miles from Lowellville, I thought I could make a go of it. I gave my two weeks' notice and left to open my own pharmacy.

I worked for six months to renovate an old building along the Mahoning River that belonged to someone else, and did so without working elsewhere as a pharmacist, so I was not generating income. County loans were available, which I took advantage of, and I foraged for whatever else I could find to finish the job. I used a sledgehammer to knock out the opening for four large windows overlooking the river, built a fountain inside, and had a nice counseling area for my customers. It was beautiful when done, with new canvas awnings over the windows, a portrait of the Lowellville Bridge painted on the side of the building, and shelves stocked with all the sundries a pharmacy needed. Unfortunately, I was too young to realize that I was about to open an independent pharmacy when their demise had all but been guaranteed by the aggressiveness of the chain pharmacy industry.

The wholesaler who stocked my pharmacy could have done me the favor of declining my application for credit, but they didn't. I would eventually owe them the difference between what they brought in as merchandise when I opened against what was left to take when I closed. I opened on October 2, 1988, and closed on January 1, 1989, and in that short period of time, I racked up $33,000 in debt to my wholesaler, I maxed out my credit cards, and I had a community improvement loan to pay back to the county.

Carlson's Riverside Pharmacy, as I dubbed it, must hold the record for the shortest-lived retail pharmacy in the history of the U.S. It opened the same day that a new and growing pharmacy chain called Phar-Mor opened their flagship store in Boardman, Ohio, just a few miles away. They deeply discounted everything, including prescription drugs, and handed out coupons and free two-liter bottles of pop to everyone who walked in. Their cool neon lights mesmerized the public. My customers in Struthers, who I thought loved me enough to make the drive to Lowellville, and the residents of Lowellville themselves didn't transfer their prescriptions to me. By the time we opened, I had already gone six months without a pharmacist's salary, I was in debt, and I was annoyed that my potential customers were being drawn away from the services I thought I could provide for nearly the same cost.

My store was only open for a few months, but it was a long enough period spent in quiet boredom to give me the impression that people were beginning to want anonymity. It wasn't the first time I'd had this epiphany, but it was the first time the thought mattered to me. Although HIPPA laws did not yet exist and mail-order pharmacy had not yet reached its peak, both were right around the corner and would, in small or big ways, add to people's solitude.

In the 2020 miniseries *The Queen's Gambit*, set in the 1950s and '60s, there's a scene in which the protagonist, Beth, interacts with a pharmacist. The pharmacist pulls down his glasses to give her a stern look before he agrees to fill a prescription for her mother. When he returns to the counter to hand Beth her mother's prescription, he issues a warning to pass a long about the number of days the prescription should last. The pharmacist knew Beth's mother, was aware of her drug use, and gave a police-like impression that he would not tolerate signs of abuse. He had rightfully participated in the system of checks and balances meant to protect his public from misusing the drugs he dispensed.

This historical pharmacy expectation of necessary human interactions between pharmacist and patient still existed in 1988, but it was beginning to be pushed aside by prescription volume and non-pharmacy related gimmicks. The checks-and-balances role of the pharmacist with physician that was being ignored by chain pharmacies was allowing anonymity to exist in an industry that had laws forbidding it. Drugs, not bread, was the article of commerce being sold. When this lawful expectation of a pharmacist is ignored and anonymity takes its place, we allow abuses and addictions to feed the very behavior that leads to our desire for anonymity in the first place. Patient information needs to be shared with professionals—who should themselves demand it when the law requires it.

Looking back, the business side of my pharmacy didn't get off to a good start, and my hormones were partially to blame. Yes, it was a beautiful store, and the grand opening was celebrated with the Lowellville Mt. Carmel Club Band and Mayor Rossi and I making speeches in front of TV cameras, with my proud parents looking on. I'm glad I captured it all with my camcorder. Well, almost all. I didn't record my late arrival. I slept in after enjoying a night on the town with the beautiful Lori Bisconti. All the work I had put into opening my very own pharmacy was jeopardized by a twenty-six-year-old's gland that saw nothing but beauty. Lori had been working as a waitress at Geno's Restaurant across the street, and I went in there almost daily for rigatoni and meatballs, always hoping that she was working and assigned to my seating area.

She was and still is the queen bee of Lowellville. She is strong and determined, confident and beautiful, and has sacrificed some of herself to make others what they could be. She continues to be the rock upon which I, our children, and our relatives and friends stand.

I was in love, in debt, and bitter that my store was failing due to the lack of love the community was showing me. My propensity to throw financial caution to the wind finally served me well the day I reached into the cash register and emptied it of all its money. I put an "Out of business" sign on the door and drove to the jewelers to purchase an engagement ring. My life was moving quickly and dramatically now that I had met that special someone, and I would leave my first old building remodel and my failed pharmacy in the rearview mirror.

After my store closed, I went back to work for Revco with my tail between my legs. Eighteen months later, in 1990, Lori and I were married. It was a beautiful ceremony held in Holy Rosary Church of Lowellville, with a very large Italian reception following. On our honeymoon, we sat at a kitchen table in a condominium in Ocean City, Maryland, and saw all the gifts of money we received from the 750-plus guests at our wedding go out the door to pay my bills. That, I am confident, was her idea.

◆ ◆ ◆

5
THE OHIO PHARMACISTS ASSOCIATION

In 1989, while Lori and I were dating, I was fixing up my brother's old house, working three jobs to pay back my debts, and struggling to make good on commitments I'd previously made to professional pharmacy associations. After graduating from ONU in May of 1985 and having served as our college representative to the Ohio Pharmacists Association, a professional association that represents all pharmacists in Ohio, I ran for second vice-president of OPA after the executive director of the association, Phil Cramer, Esq. suggested that I do so. This office, if won, would eventually progress to first vice-president, then president-elect, and eventually president. It was a bold and confident move so soon after graduation that probably no one had made before. Still, I had just finished several years of intense association participation, and I felt I would be ready to wield the gavel of such a large organization. After all, I would have three years to prepare, and I was young and uncommitted.

Phil Cramer seemed to like me, or so I thought. I should have listened to the officers of our county's local association and turned him down, but instead, I drove to Columbus where he and I formulated a campaign strategy and wrote letters. It was an awkward day at the OPA office, full of strange conversations and heated exchanges, and I drove home thinking that I was being used for something other than my ability to lead an organization. A fight was brewing among members of OPA, and Phil's push for me to run for office had more to do with keeping someone else from having the office. At the age of twenty-four, I was being looked at as a puppet that was not capable of doing harm to some future agenda they had.

Ignorance is bliss when a newly licensed pharmacist believes they can lead without any practical pharmacy knowledge at all, and I was ignorant. I knew nothing about Medicaid or Worker's Compensation issues, the plight of independent pharmacies, the rise of mail-order pharmacy, or how prescription drugs were priced. Were it not for a division brewing under the surface between two factions of leaders, I would not have won. I was unaware of this rift that had the Board of Trustees and officers taking sides and dividing their votes. In the end, many votes were cast for me only because they were opposed to another who was running for the same office. I won the election by a narrow margin, and had been successfully used to pull votes away from another candidate. If I'd known anything about the fight being waged behind the scenes or the fight yet to come, I would have declined his suggestion to run when we first spoke. In this case, my true lack of knowledge and experience placed me in a difficult position. We all have things in life we wish we could do over again; this is one of mine.

The timing was bad for me because I had just closed a failed pharmacy, I was about to get married, my parents had just moved to Florida, and I was in debt. My position with OPA came with several perks, though, and one was that Revco Drug was quick to take me back after my store closed. Unfortunately, before that, McKesson

Drug, my wholesaler, had apparently thought that the president of OPA was a sure-enough bet to extend me a great deal of credit for my store in the form of all that merchandise. I was spending beyond my means. Credit cards were becoming a thing at the time, and going into debt was easy for those who didn't take the time to flip over the statements that revealed in fine print the interest rates attached to their spending. I was riding nearly $50,000 of debt, and in 1989, that was a lot of money.

I don't know how I managed to stay afloat financially, but I did—and without hurting my credit score. All I can say is that I'm a worker. I was able to tread water well enough in most areas of my life to get by, even though it felt like things were moving at the speed of light.

But then, it was time for me to assume the office of president of OPA, and it happened a bit sooner than I wanted. I was young, debt-ridden, and trapped in the stresses associated with working retail chain pharmacy. To make matters worse, the association's officers and board members were still fighting among themselves, resigning, or being fired. Welcome to the world of professional associations. I was young, and because of the resignations and firings, had to assume the role of president of OPA a year sooner that I was supposed to.

I always read the governing documents of an organization before taking on a leadership role within it, and OPA was no exception. The truth can almost always be found in an organization's constitution and bylaws. They clarify ambiguities, establish order, allow for the expression of ideas, and rein in those who believe they can function outside it. There was nowhere else for me to turn during the short period of time that I had to ready myself except the constitution and bylaws of OPA, so I studied these guiding principles and sorted through the various sections to gain a better understanding of the organization—and perhaps avoid embarrassment for having accepted the responsibility before I was truly ready.

In the mid-1980s, computer technology was just emerging onto the scene, and I turned to it, even though I could ill-afford it. I purchased the new toy on the market known as a home computer. It was an IBM PC Jr., and it seemed like more of a digital typewriter than anything else. If you could figure out how to save data at all, it was stored on floppy disks, which were plastic disks encased in paper envelopes that were inserted and ejected—if they ejected at all. Less than 20 percent of American households had a personal home computer at the time, and that rarity made it difficult to set up and use. You couldn't simply take it out of the box, plug it in, and follow a few simple instructions for firing it up. It was a heavy machine with a TV screen for a monitor and a thick operator's manual. It was another debt-financed purchase, like my camcorder, that I rationalized away as an investment. In spite of the high cost at the time and the limitations it had, the computer's ability to backspace, erasing words, and then rewrite without using Wite-Out or tossing the page completely was a godsend. I had a copy of OPA's constitution and bylaws, and I got busy typing it all onto a floppy disk.

I spent weeks trying to figure out who the important OPA players were, who oversaw what, who answered to whom, and how to remove a rogue executive director of a state pharmacists association without a breach of contract claim coming back to bite us. I now needed to cut ties with the man who helped me get elected, and the means of doing so was somewhere in these governing documents.

My first year as an elected officer was spent listening to the toxic bickering that sometimes is necessary to start anew. Low and behold, and in the midst of this bickering, I stood up at a meeting and cited the section of our OPA bylaws that would allow us to remove Phil without worrying that he would come back with a breach of contract claim. So much for the kid who could do no harm. We succeeded in firing Phil. Afterward, many on the board resigned, including an officer ahead of me. This meant that I would become president a year sooner than I had anticipated, and although I was still ignorant of many pharmacy issues, I was at least familiar with the organization's founding documents and guidelines.

OPA represents all pharmacists in Ohio, and certain association activities cannot be misconstrued to favor one practice setting over another. As mentioned earlier, OPA had formed a GPO to help independent pharmacists, and although this may not be disallowed, the association had engaged in activities that went against the totality of representation that OPA is bound to uphold. After Phil's removal, our search committee met and selected someone to take his place: Ernie Boyd, R.Ph. Ernie stepped down a few weeks ago. Many pharmacists across the country know of OPA's accomplishments under his direction, and I consider myself fortunate to have been an OPA president during his tenure. He helped this very young man survive a role that was meant for someone more seasoned, and I will always be grateful to him for his assistance.

I remember parts of the speech I gave the night I was installed as president, but it was getting up from my seat at the head table and walking to the podium that I remember most. The last time I stood up in front of a crowded room of professionals, I fell flat on my face; not so this time. My OPA president's speech referenced the beauty of an old building and how things were constructed in the "old days" when we took the time to create beauty by paying attention to the details. Our details were in the form of the rules established when the association was founded, and our best hope for success would be in gathering as many people as possible to the cause and following the rules as outlined or collectively changing them if they were outdated. It's possible that I compared these things to the beauty of an old building because I had just finished renovating a couple of my own. I didn't embarrass myself this time, and another gavel was handed to me, beginning what I can only now characterize as a youthful blur from which I would take away pieces of a bigger picture.

I assumed the role of a president of a state pharmacy association at the record age of twenty-seven. That record stands today in the U.S. I carried the anxiety of unknown situations, along with my own financial limitations, to places I didn't belong at that age. This prevented me from being the type of president I needed to be, especially given what our profession was beginning to face.

At one point, I was invited to speak to the local association in Cleveland, one of the largest groups in the state, and I spent weeks preparing my talk. I laid out on overhead transparencies an explanation of OPA's constitution and bylaws, the beauty and simplicity of the writings of previous leaders, and the potential our pharmacy profession could realize if we embraced them. I knew this subject well and was prepared for the talk. The only problem was that I thought I was speaking on a Thursday and the meeting was on a Wednesday. There were no cell phones in 1989, no text messages to serve as reminders, only landline phones that would ring the next day to tell you what you'd missed. I was embarrassed that I had stood them up and disappointed my friend Alva Rubenstein, R.Ph. and upset that I was unable to deliver the presentation I had worked so hard to prepare.

We can sulk about these things and wish they'd never happened, or we can appreciate the experience and what it has given us. Despite my youthful shortcomings, I believe that my experiences with professional association leadership made me a better person, pharmacist, and leader. Just as I had taken lessons from my time at

ONU, I would take from OPA what I needed to help me do better in the future. Yes, I made some missteps, but I also taught myself the workings of professional associations and additional rules contained in Ohio law.

Somewhere in a box on a shelf is a VHS tape with a recording of a local association meeting that Ernie and I spoke at during my tenure as president. I recorded the discussions that independent pharmacists were having about the rise of mail-order pharmacies and the impact it was beginning to have on their ability to compete. The emergence of mail-order pharmacies marked the beginning of the end for independent pharmacy as we knew it. We had no way of seeing into the future, but if we had even a glimpse of the impact mail-order pharmacy and chain pharmacy would eventually have on patient care, prescription costs, or independent pharmacy, we would have raised our voices much louder—and perhaps even screamed. My debt-funded camcorder was an investment in documenting history.

In 1989, I was once again working for the retail chain Revco and driving fifty minutes from my home in Canfield to Ravenna each day. Each Revco store had a number, and the Ravenna store, #1303, was known as "The Zoo." It was a very busy store both behind the pharmacy counter and out front on the OTC floor. I had not yet been exposed to high prescription volumes, and store #1303 had one pharmacist filling over three hundred prescriptions a day. The citizens of Ravenna purchased just about everything the store had to offer, to the point where the regional Revco saying was, "If you can't sell it at your store, put it on the truck to Ravenna, and they'll sell it."

The type of customer connection I had enjoyed while working at the Revco in Struthers just wasn't possible at the Revco in Ravenna.

It was much too busy and a far cry from the environment I'd enjoyed previously or had expected to enjoy when graduating from college. I needed to work at this store for only a few short weeks to know that a place like Carlson's Riverside Pharmacy was never going to work in this day and age. I had walked into a different type of pharmacy practice, and I did not like it. The days were long and full of hustle. There were no breaks, I was on my feet twelve to thirteen hours a day, and on the drive home, I often had that hypertensive feeling in my brain caused by massive reductions in serotonin levels.

Eventually, dispensing a controlled substance to a patient is what prompted me to give my two weeks' notice. For months, I had been dispensing brand-name Percocet, a narcotic for treating pain, for a man who always sent his wife (red flag) to have it filled. He never wanted the cheaper generic (red flag), and his wife showed up like clockwork on the thirtieth day for his refill (another red flag), so I became suspicious and confronted his wife. She was a shy, timid person, but when I questioned her, she explained the situation. Her husband worked for an electrical contractor and was on the back of a truck when its breaks released and backed into a power line. The electrical current traveled down the boom and continued through the truck. He lost both arms that were holding onto the truck (the entry point for the current) and a leg (the exit point) and suffered burns over most of his body. I backed away, felt relieved that she had not taken offense, and cursed myself for the volume-driven insensitivity I had allowed to develop within me. Patient care was changing in pharmacy, and I had just been bitten by it.

I planned my escape from The Zoo soon thereafter. Before leaving, I set up my camcorder on a tripod and recorded a day's worth of activity. I'm not sure what explanation I gave at the time, but no one seemed to think anything of it. The professional side of me knew something was wrong with the way this store was filling prescriptions, it was becoming more commonplace within the chain and among my colleagues with whom I frequently conversed, and I wanted to get it on tape. I had no intentions of using it in support of any radical actions of mine. I just wanted to capture it for my own sake.

◆ ◆ ◆

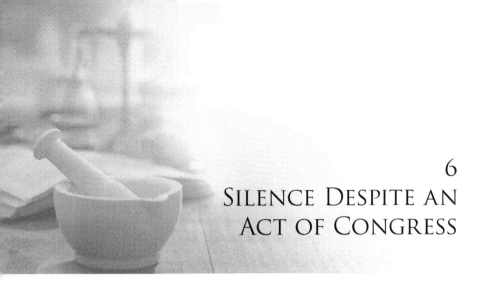

6
SILENCE DESPITE AN
ACT OF CONGRESS

IT WAS DURING THE LATE 80S when the public began to sense the dangerous pace at which pharmacies, like the one I had just left, were operating. The mom-and-pop way of controlling prescription drug use by maintaining pharmacist-patient relationships (human interaction) was slowly but surely being replaced by volume and insurance distractions. More and more insurance paperwork that had once been sent off for HQ to handle was now being handled by pharmacists directly, and these monetary distractions were beginning to bog down thoughtful dispensing functions. Computers were also coming onto the scene. They could transmit data in real time, but pharmacists needed to be able to make corrections immediately. Otherwise, a prescription label couldn't be generated to put on the bottle. It was a staggering transition that was turning patients into numbers and occurred in just five years' time.

Drug dispensing that once had a component of conversation attached to it had turned into counting by fives, adjudicating insurance claims, and glancing up only when the patient was being rung up at the register to see if they were okay with the copay they were charged. To make matters worse, just when we thought we had begun to master a particular computer system, a new one was installed that would supposedly make our lives easier. We had to deal with constant new computer and phone systems, prescription-filling systems, and insurance company takeovers that gave pharmacists one insurance problem after another. Patients rarely had the correct or updated insurance cards, they were difficult to read, and each had its own set of codes that required a manual of the National Council for Prescription Drug Programs (NCPDP) that was several hundred pages long just to speak the language necessary to get a prescription claim to transmit successfully.

Pharmacists were becoming insurance agents while still having to maintain control of drug distribution. Traditionally, "control" meant interacting with the person you were about to hand drugs to. By having some level of human interaction with a patient and knowing who they were and what their condition was, a pharmacist could dispense drugs with a certain measure of confidence that those drugs would "do no harm." This is the best and safest way a pharmacist can know if they are dispensing the right drug for the right patient, making them less likely to experience adverse drug reactions. It's an important responsibility that is difficult to adhere to when a pharmacist has been turned into a hurried insurance agent. Everyone knew it, except those who didn't want to. What we all should have known—and what eventually came back to bite the public—was that our hurried pace prevented us from determining a legitimate prescription from one that was not. Instead, it seemed more important to determine a legitimate insurance customer from one who was not.

The corporate owners of chain pharmacies learned how to "bicker" for insurance contracts so they could gain customers. They would win exclusive contracts with large employers by bidding down the amount of money they would accept from that employer's insurance company in exchange for dispensing a prescription, called a dispensing fee. As a result, millions of patients were no longer able to have their prescriptions filled at the independent stores they had developed a relationship with. CVS, for example, would bid $3.00 to dispense a drug for, say, all employees working at General Motors. Rite Aid would counter with a bid of $2.50. Walgreens lowered the fee by bidding $2.00, and Walmart would win it with $1.50. The race to the bottom was underway.

The pace quickened at chain pharmacies when customers were "incentivized" to transfer their prescriptions away from the independent pharmacies that served them. The chain pharmacists now had to absorb the customer base of those independent pharmacies, and the salaries of those who now had to work faster climbed disproportionately to other professions at the time. And just as one would expect, the race to the bottom did not escape public notice, even though few paid attention to yet another boarded-up building in Smalltown, U.S.A., that once housed an independent pharmacy.

Reports of hospitalizations due to misuse of prescription drugs were beginning to surface as data-driven computers became increasingly common. Furthermore, the increased costs associated with drug-related admissions caught the attention of the U.S. government, which was financially frugal at the time. One remedy involved legally defining the role of the pharmacist. Clearly, citizens must have thought they weren't getting their money's worth or lawmakers suspected that danger lurked, because our profession was about to become subject to a one-thousand-page law, which it had earned.

Congress proposed an act to rein in these moral hazards and dictate what a pharmacist was legally required to do when dispensing prescription drugs to the public. The American Pharmacists Association—along with individual state pharmacy associations—saw the disparity between pharmacists' professional obligations and real-world practices, and they supported its passage. Except for the National Association of Chain Drug Stores (NACDS), most pharmacy organizations endorsed the law because it offered a definition for our profession, and expectations about an important social role that could not be easily taken from us. We now knew who we were and what we were supposed to do.

On November 5, 1990, The Omnibus Reconciliation Act (OBRA-90) became law. A portion of that law, Drug Use Review (DUR) was intended to reduce government spending on prescription drugs by requiring pharmacists to assume specific responsibilities with "each and every" prescription dispensed. This federal law was to encourage pharmacists to use reasonable care in three main areas of pharmacy practice: when the prescription is handed to the pharmacist, when the prescription is filled, and when the prescription drugs are handed to the patient. Being a federal law, states were given three years to pass their own laws to ensure compliance if they wanted to received federal funds.

Note: addiction is an adverse drug reaction.

Please see **Addendum 1** to read the text of OBRA-90, Drug Use Review, but here is a condensed version—an opioid-relevant version—of what the law requires:

FEDERAL: AS PASSED BY CONGRESS AND SIGNED INTO LAW ON NOVEMBER 5, 1990

a. H.R. 5835 (101st): Omnibus Budget Reconciliation Act of 1990 (OBRA-90)
(g) DRUG USE REVIEW-

—States have until January 1, 1993 to provide a program that assures prescriptions are: appropriate, medically necessary, and not likely to result in adverse drug reactions.

—States have until January 1, 1993 to provide a program that monitors pharmacists and physicians and identifies patterns of fraud, abuse, gross overuse, and unnecessary care.

—States shall require their pharmacists to perform Drug Utilization Review (DUR) before a drug is dispensed to a patient. The review shall look for abuse/misuse and inappropriate lengths of time that patients use prescription drugs. Pharmacists shall screen for drug problems (addiction), duplication of similar drugs from one or more physicians, and drug interactions.

—States shall recognize the importance of a pharmacist providing counseling to patients by asking that the pharmacist personally offer to discuss in person:

◆ name and description of the drug

◆ how it's to be taken and for how long it's to be taken

◆ special directions

◆ what side effects or adverse effects (addiction) a patient could experience

◆ how a patient can avoid serious reactions

- how the patient might know if the drug is helping or harming them

- how to store the drug

- whether the prescription could or should be refilled

- what a patient should do if they miss taking a dose

—States shall require pharmacists to make a "reasonable effort" to find out who a patient is, what is wrong with them, why they are having a prescription filled and keep the information current in the patient's record:

- patient name, address, phone number, date of birth, and gender

- a list of the medications currently being taken

- allergies a patient might have to drugs

- list of over-the-counter medications

- any previous adverse reactions (addiction/allergy) a patient has had

- the disease or diseases from which they suffer

- any medical devices a patient my be using (pacemaker, catheter, insulin pump, C-Pap machine for sleep apnea, hearing aids, contacts lens, implanted heart defibrillator, walkers, wheel chair, braces, oxygen, colostomy bag, etc.)

- a record of personal comments made by a pharmacist that is relevant to any patient information he/she received when the prescriptions were dropped off, problems they saw when they considered whether or not to dispense the drug to the patient, and pertinent information they either gave or received from a patient when personally counseling them.

—States do not have to require pharmacists to counsel if patients sign away their rights that would have required them to do so.

—States shall establish a Drug Use Review Board made up of pharmacists and physicians to:

- look at prescribing data and dispensing data to identify trends that raise red flags of abuse and misuse of prescription drugs.

- intervene with physicians and pharmacists if problems with drug therapy are identified and use intense intervention if individual physicians and pharmacists are identified as problems.

- after intervening with physicians and pharmacists who appear to be creating drug-use problems, wait a while and see if the intervention has worked.

- remind physicians and pharmacists of their duties if they have neglected them, remind them of their powers if they

have discounted them, and provide each with those acceptable standards by which they are expected to practice.

+ provide an annual report of its finding to the Secretary so
someone higher up could act if action was thought necessary.

+ the Secretary shall read the report and determine if each
state's Drug Use program is effective in preventing the drug-
use problems that OBRA-90 was enacted to prevent.

The purpose of OBRA-90 was to thwart the abuse and misuse
of prescription drugs, almost as if the people had a premonition of
the coming opioid addiction epidemic. It was meant to define the
care a pharmacist needed to provide before handing a dangerous
drug to a citizen. The law instructed pharmacists to slow down,
gather information, make educated decisions, document concerns,
and converse with the patient so they knew the importance of the
drug they were about to consume. This checklist of pharmacists'
responsibilities is supposed to be completed before patients take
possession of the drug, not after.

In Ohio, our citizens thought that OBRA-90 and Drug Use Review
were of such importance that our Board of Pharmacy made its rules
mandatory for all prescriptions filled, not just those paid for with
federal dollars. It didn't matter if you were a Medicaid patient or
not; the federal OBRA-90 law and the subsequent rules passed by
our Ohio Board of Pharmacy would safeguard everyone in Ohio from
unsafe dispensing practices.

Prior to the 1993 deadline, the Ohio BOP passed specific rules
to which a pharmacist must adhere when engaging in the practice
of pharmacy in the state of Ohio. State laws are contained in the

Ohio Revised Code (ORC), and the rules that various agencies write are found in the Ohio Administrative Code (OAC). As you will read, OAC is much more specific than the corresponding Federal OBRA-90.

These are Ohio's rules, though most other states' rules are similar. Please read Addendum 2 for the full text, but here is a condensed version—an opioid relevant version—of what the rules require:

THE OHIO ADMINISTRATIVE CODE, AS CONTAINED IN OAC 4729-5-21, MANNER OF PROCESSING A PRESCRIPTION, REQUIRES THE FOLLOWING:

—prescriptions are not valid if they are not prescribed for a legitimate medical purpose.

—pharmacists are just as responsible as physicians in making sure that illegitimate prescription drugs are not dispensed to patients.

—an illegitimate prescription is an order for a drug that is outside the scope of a "bona fide" treatment.

—a pharmacist who knowingly dispenses an illegitimate prescription is subject to the penalities of law just as the physician is who prescribed it.

—before handing a prescription drug to a patient, a pharmacist must ensure that he/she knows certain information about the patient, that the drug is safe for that patient to take, it is labeled correctly, the patient is offered to be counseled so as to be informed of the dangers of that drug, and information obtained when dispensing the drug is placed on record.

—a pharmacist must make a reasonable attempt to obtain all the patient information that is required in OBRA-90: name, address, DOB, etc.

—a pharmacist must take the necessary time to review whether the prescription is appropriate (legitimate) based on the patient information that was received from the patient and either accept or reject the prescription before placing drug in a bottle and affixing a label.

—if a pharmacist spots and potential problems, he/she is to resolve the problem and place a note in the patient's profile as to what he/she did.

—a pharmacist is to enter notes that are unique to the patient and the drug therapy being prescribed.

—physicians are responsible for proper prescribing, but pharmacists are equally responsible for determining whether a prescription is for a legitimate medical purpose or not.

—a pharmacist does not have to dispense a drug if he/she thinks it is not for a legitimate medical purpose.

—a pharmacist shall have the freedom to use his/her professional judgment.

—a pharmacist or designee shall personally offer the services of prescription counseling.

—a pharmacist shall discuss with the patient all that is required in OBRA-90.

—a patient is allowed to sign away their right to receive this important information if they wish, and if they know what it is they are signing.

Despite these federal and state regulations, in the ensuing years, chain pharmacies would read between the lines of this law, examine the gray areas, disregard the people's intentions, and otherwise bend or skirt the law to accommodate the number of prescriptions they won through the contracts they signed, the promotions they offered, or the discounts that bankrupted their independent pharmacy competitors. And all the while, chain pharmacists remained silent in exchange for their salaries. It was corporate fertilizer, combined with expensive pharmacist tears, that fed and watered the seeds that eventually grew into an epidemic.

Given all the personal interaction, professional consideration, and patient documentation required by this law, anyone reading it would have to wonder how it was possible that the addictive property of OxyContin could go undetected for as long as it did. Notwithstanding any failed laboratory tests, skewed documents, or failed FDA oversight, how could we not have seen it in the eyes of our patients or read the concerns of other pharmacists in profile notes? Was there no eye contact? Were there no notes for pharmacists to consult and recognize patterns of addiction? And if there was a pattern, did pharmacists not take steps to verify their suspicions? Who or what was preventing the exchange of information between pharmacist and patient or between pharmacists themselves?

Simply put, the law says to be on the lookout for addiction, which is referred to as "abuse" or "misuse." Addiction is one of the most recognizable adverse drug reactions to spot. Addiction is a side effect, not a disease, and it should have been detected as such. Each time a patient wanted another refill of OxyContin, they had to obtain a new prescription from their physician and present it to the pharmacist because it is a Schedule II drug. Automatic refills are not allowed for such drugs, and a new prescription must be presented for each fill. The "manner of processing a prescription," which each pharmacist had to adhere to, applied each time. A prescription drug that is allowed one year's worth of refills could fly under the radar much more easily than a drug like Percocet, Fentanyl, or OxyContin, since there are twelve opportunities to engage with a patient instead of one. So, how did we not see this greatest of adverse effects if the law was enacted specifically to allow us to do just that? Clearly, we weren't following the law as intended.

Our profession and our pharmacists have been held hostage by business models that have driven the slow creep away from what was written in 1990. One moral hazard after another was added by corporate pharmacy and was done so in a way that it escaped everyone's attention. They installed drive-thru windows, knowing that no one would want to sit in their idle car, wasting gas as they divulge endless personal secrets or listen to twenty-one facts about a drug when they can just read a pamphlet or search the internet. When they sign for their prescription, almost no one will read the fine print and notice that they have declined their right to be counseled.

Board of Pharmacy agents do not typically inspect patient profiles to see if pharmacists are taking the time to type notes in a patient's profile that are "pertinent to drug therapy," so they never noticed that the drug counseling logs showed that patients were declining their right to be counseled 95 percent of the time. Give the "customer" a coupon if there is a dispensing error, and you ensure that they never see themselves as patients, sue for damages, or notify the Board of Pharmacy. Give pharmacy technicians the code to override computer warnings when they pop up, and staff will never see themselves as healthcare providers.

Federal and state law is sometimes vague because legislators like to leave the dirty work of writing the specific language to agencies. These organizations form a de facto fourth branch of government whose employees are not elected and who cannot be voted out of office, and yet, their power is immense. Yes, directors of agencies can be fired if an elected leader decides to relieve them of their duties. But that usually takes a huge effort, and short of that, the public is too far removed from a process of accountability to institute change when the system fails to function as laws had intended it to. It is agencies that define the intent of the law, and in Ohio's case, the Ohio Board of Pharmacy was very specific in the rules it wrote, interpreting what the people specifically intended when they passed federal OBRA-90.

With OBRA-90 on the books, pharmacists had a legal manual to follow that would prevent drug misuse, and not only would the people be spared from the suffering of misuse, they would enjoy seeing the reduction in prescription drug costs that the law was also meant to address. But in reality, pharmacists did not follow the law as intended. They gathered only basic information from patients, they were not given time to thoughtfully consider DUR, and almost everyone declined patient counseling. This is what we were seeing in 1990 when OBRA-90 was passed. And aside from some changes that corporate computer geeks made to our prescription filling systems, the only implementation we pharmacists saw was a signature log placed on the checkout counter for patients to sign away their right to be counseled by a pharmacist.

Corporate pharmacy tacitly encouraged rule-bending, and apathetic chain pharmacists allowed the rules to be broken. Chain pharmacists allowed a workplace environment that gathered only a patient's name, address, phone number, and birthdate during initial screening instead of the twelve pieces of information suggested by the law. They sped through the DUR in six seconds instead of the six minutes suggested by the law. They were okay with patients walking out of pharmacies thinking they had signed their names to verify for their insurance companies that they had received the drug and not that they had signed away their right to be counseled. After all, who would ask: "The pharmacist would like to talk to you about twenty important things you should know before taking this medication" when "Do you have any questions for the pharmacist?" is more conducive to a fast paced corporate business model.

Deceptive corporate business models went unchallenged by pharmacists who stubbornly clung to professional apathy. They would accept their working conditions in exchange for high salaries, complain to one another privately instead of working together, and fail to leverage their importance in a pharmacist shortage to demand change. They turned their backs on the public by not collectively challenging the business models that brought daily complaints, and none of them wanted to or intentionally meant to. I know I didn't, and I was working in the trenches with them at the time. Every single one of us would rather have been given the time to sit down with patients and use the education we had worked hard and long to obtain. This was not possible. We were being told what to do by employers who believed that time was endlessly available to us.

During the early years of abuse by their corporate employers, chain pharmacists' complaints could be characterized by the term "kicking the cat." Pharmacists would go home each night after a busy twelve-hour day and complain to their spouse, who would in turn complain about something to their child. Eventually, the totality of the frustration would be relieved when the child complained to the pet cat by kicking it. This was how the food chain of complaints went. There was nothing concrete, nothing signed in protest, and certainly no organized attempts by chain pharmacists to address their professional downward slide. Other established pharmacy organizations in other practice settings (independent, hospital, consulting) sensed the dangers and knew that their colleagues were irresponsibly handing out drugs, and yet, it continued unabated without any concrete conversation or action. The gorilla of unprofessionalism was left sitting in the corner as though it never existed.

Salaries continued to climb higher and higher, especially when compared with other professions, and pharmacy technicians, who were being equally abused by the system, made about one-fifth a pharmacist's wage. Still, the shortage of pharmacists within the profession meant that a pharmacist could threaten to quit if they felt professionally violated or believed that public safety was at risk. Since there was no one to hire in their place, playing that card could have been very effective and brought about change quickly. Unfortunately, few did.

The handsome salaries that put pharmacists in the top 10 percent of wage earners worked as effectively as lashes from a whip when corporate owners wanted their bricks made without straw. This prevented any coordinated efforts to change the status quo, no matter how much workplace pain resulted for pharmacists or how much death and disease from drug misuse and dispensing errors befell the public. The chain pharmacist was, essentially, being paid off. Most would have gladly exchanged the money that was being thrown at them for more help, fewer distractions, and additional time to comply with the humane world of dispensing that OBRA-90 had just offered them. Instead, corporate chain pharmacies read the law and wondered how they might get around it instead of embracing it for the patient safety it offered the public and the sanity it offered its pharmacists.

◆ ◆ ◆

7
SOUNDS LIKE A
PHARMACIST'S UNION

EVERYTHING MEANINGFUL IN THE CONSTITUTION and bylaws
of the various professional pharmacy organizations I had been
involved with was missing from the life of the chain pharmacist, and
in 1990, I was still working for the chain Revco Drug. I was a chain
pharmacist myself and felt totally alone. There was no single organization for chain pharmacists at the state or national level. Because
of this, there were no complaints, concerns, ideas, or camaraderie
with others in my situation. There was no chain representative to
apply pressure to the powers in charge, no magazines specific to our
practice setting, no officers we could elect to speak on our behalf,
nothing! All we had at our disposal to relieve our frustration was
to kick the cat.

And this was not a small, insignificant practice setting. Chain
pharmacists account for over 60 percent of the profession, dwarfing
all the others combined. With more than 230,000 educated chain
professionals who, in the early 1980s, contributed to pharmacy being
ranked near the top in each year's Gallop polls of most trusted profession, our country's democratic void was big.

Those who understand the inherent benefits of democracy and its ability to keep the wolves at bay could see that the immense drug-dispensing activity happening at the hands of chain pharmacists lacked the essential ingredient of democracy that, in my opinion, would be the underlying cause of our nation's drug misuse. Nothing was said about dangerous working conditions because chain pharmacists denied themselves the ability to say it existed. They represented the majority of pharmacists that were handing prescription drugs to patients and yet they were the only practice setting that did not have an organization to represent their interests.

I ended my term as OPA president wondering where all the chain pharmacists were. Few joined the organization, and among those who did, the number that attended organization meetings was pathetic. For years, this fact dominated my thoughts. This imbalance was my most important takeaway from OPA, and from then on, I deemed this Issue #1.

I saw the apathy of the chain pharmacist as the biggest threat to public safety, and I did not have an answer as to why or how it existed. How could the largest practice setting in such a socially important profession be without a single professional organization to represent it, when the other pharmaceutical settings had over 250? Was it the money? Was it fear of retaliation? Apathy? Had no one ever thought to organize one? Maybe they thought that the National Association of Chain Drug Stores (NACDS) was an organization they could join, and never realized it was a trade association of chain owners? I gave these chain pharmacists the benefit of the doubt and believed that I had just stumbled upon a novel idea to help pharmacy that no one had thought of. I would take it upon myself to organize a professional association to represent chain pharmacists.

Although one could now say that my impulsiveness has served me well over the years, that certainly was not the case when I gave Revco my two-week notice. I should have stayed in spite of the difficult pace I had to work, but I had grown tired of the fifty minute drive, and a close call twice on the interstate with tractor-trailer rigs convinced me that I needed to work closer to home. Pharmacist jobs were everywhere, and it seemed to be a foregone conclusion that I could find another in just a day or two; everyone was able to at that time.

I had one big problem while working at Revco Drug in Ravenna and noticing the dangerous path pharmacy was heading. So after having just finished my presidency of OPA that showed the absence of chain pharmacists, I began testing the waters to form a national association to represent chain pharmacists. In 1991, I started to run my mouth and pass out literature to my fellow chain pharmacists about joining an organization that I was trying to get off the ground. I called it the National Association of Employee Pharmacists (NAEP), and because it sounded like a union, I was unable to find a new job, despite there being a shortage of pharmacists. I was a good pharmacist, and my interviews seemed to go well, but I wasn't hired anywhere.

The work I was doing to get this "first of a kind" chain pharmacist association off the ground was done by snail mail and phone calls, and although the word would spread much slower than through today's use of the internet, it was fast enough to place a label on me in my hometown. Chain pharmacies had openings minutes from my home, were giving signing bonuses, and forgiving student debt. There were pharmacists behind their counters who, like my Uncle Ray, were working into their eighties. The early 90s was a smorgasbord for anyone who had the intials R.Ph. after their name, and here

I was starving because I had Director, EOPA after mine. I should have stayed at Revco and waited for a transfer closer to home, but it never seemed to come for one reason or another, and perhaps my self-imposed unemployment only saved them from doing what they might have eventually done anyway?

I would have to find employment outside my area and away from the jibber-jabber I had created within my pharmacy circle. Why? Because a professional association acts much like a union. The two function in nearly the same way except that one requires dues, and the other does not. But as much as pharmacy employers fear the formation of a union, to me, a professional association was a more effective way to create change than a union. Congresspeople gravitate toward professional associations for the good they symbolize, and at one time, pharmacists liked to put these associations on their resumes. It was the sort of thing a good obituary was made of.

In fact, at the time, I detested the thought of a pharmacists' union and the picketing that might withhold needed medication from citizens. I thought I was working for a good and civil way to fix pharmacy's retail chain problem by offering the same type of representative voice that every other practice setting seemed to have. Only our largest setting—retail chain pharmacy—lacked one, and I thought that garnishing that immense power and affluence to further professionalism was a good thing for our profession.

Cleveland was beyond the regular earshot of my circle, and I found a job in that area. It was an hour-and-a-half from my home in sometimes brutal interstate traffic. I was newly married and living in Canfield, with a child on the way. By now, I was becoming proficient in using my home computer as a word processor, and although there was no internet yet, I began my campaign to fix dispensing issues by bringing proper representation to chain pharmacists. Unfortunately, no one told me that it would be a bad idea to pass out propaganda, especially when that propaganda sounded like an effort to organize a union.

This was the only job I was ever fired from, and the fault was solely my own. I was working at a very busy store with one other pharmacist to cover the hours and a few technicians. The pace was very fast, yet it didn't prevent me from bringing my typewriter to work. My passion for forming NAEP superseded the attention I should have been paying to my dispensing duties. I believed that I was a good judge of my use of time, and the breaks I spent typing didn't seem to interfere with my dispensing. Until it did. With my head in an NAEP cloud, I made a critical dispensing error. I gave a patient 240 milligrams of Calan SR to take three times a day instead of 250 milligrams of Ceclor. I had given someone a calcium channel blocker for the heart instead of a needed antibiotic, and that mistake landed my patient in the hospital. All I could do was sign the resignation form my supervisor placed in front of me, remove my license from the wall, and make the long walk to the front door.

I remembered nothing about the prescription I had filled in error. It had my signature, so I was the official dispenser, but like most prescriptions we filled, I never met the patient, never received any information about him prior to dispensing, didn't take the necessary time to think before bottling, and didn't counsel him before he was rung out. With or without my typewriter—which I didn't even have with me the day I committed this critical error—there was little time for the duties that would have prevented this error.

Yes, I had made a terrible error, and I owned it, but was it mine alone or did the corporate business model I was working in share some of the blame? I wasn't the only pharmacist who ever made such a dispensing error, and the fact that errors were not reported must have meant that mine was not an isolated incident. I never heard anything else about this incident from the Ohio Board of Pharmacy or any other organization, and I never found out what happened to the patient whom I harmed. I didn't add my brief stint at this location to my resume due to the unprofessional shame I felt over the situation.

It was the only mistake of this kind I would ever make.

I sobbed on the long drive home. While sitting on the stairs in our house in Canfield, I told my wife, Lori, that I had been let go. She was incredibly supportive. I suspect I misheard her kind words of "Everything is going to be okay" as "It's okay to keep going with everything."

Now I needed to find another job. My misguided confidence, along with my underestimation of chain pharmacist apathy, made me think that I didn't need to work behind a pharmacy counter at all. I could get my NAEP organization up and running and draw my income from serving as the executive director—or so I timidly tried to explain to Lori. There were 230,000 licensed chain pharmacists in the U.S. at the time; surely, a significant number of them would be interested in joining. Since our wedding funds had relieved "our" financial burdens to some extent, maybe I could give this a try.

Once the trauma of my dispensing error wore off, I was right back to working on NAEP with a new "look at what can happen because of working conditions" attitude. I was unemployed when there was an abundance of jobs in my area, I had a newborn to provide for, and yet I felt compelled to follow this path of professional association. It remains a sticking point in arguments with Lori to this day.

It was clear that technology had not yet advanced enough to help me organize quickly and efficiently. Everything was done by snail mail back then, and the wait for a reply was excruciatingly slow. I couldn't simply press a button and instantly reach hundreds or thousands of people. The times demanded that I lick thousands of envelopes in the hope that within a week or two, there would be replies with membership checks enclosed. Instead, I went to the post office to check NAEP's P.O. box each day only to be met with disappointment. Even though I tried to time my mailings so they would arrive on Fridays, when pharmacists were in their best mood, the little glass box I peered into daily told me that they were in no mood at all to hear what I had to sell them.

There were some glimmers of hope when two major pharmacy publications, *Pharmacy Times* and *Drug Topics*, published articles about NAEP and conditions behind chain pharmacy counters. These publications reached tens of thousands of pharmacists at once, and my address was clearly printed in the articles in case someone wanted additional information. But the glimmer of hope was nothing more than a prolonging of pain. The weeks that followed brought only a few notes and no money. Since time was running out with my finances, I had to ask myself how much chain pharmacist apathy must I be shown before moving on. I eventually stopped my work on NAEP and began looking for a job. I was licking envelopes containing my resume instead of pharmacy propaganda.

My father-in-law, Richard Bisconti, was a bigwig in the healthcare insurance industry and was the one who eventually signed the checks from Blue Cross to hospitals. He also chaired a committee that hospitals had to seek approval from before adding a wing or purchasing an expensive piece of equipment. This committee no longer exists, but back then, insurance companies knew that their costs would rise with hospital upgrades if those upgrades couldn't be justified, and my father-in-law was the one who decided if something was justified or not. He had the pull I needed to get back into the workplace, and he secured a job for me at St. Joseph's Hospital about forty-five minutes from my home. I was about to make a big leap from retail-chain pharmacy to hospital pharmacy, and although I knew nothing about this practice setting, I would learn quickly.

After being unemployed for four months, I began working at St. Joseph's Hospital in Warren, Ohio, in the fall of 1991, and was welcomed to the department by Dr. John Ulrich and the pharmacy staff. Sister Mildred Ely ran the hospital, and she stopped by to say hello on my first day of work. I wasted no time cleaning and organizing the back room as a way of familiarizing myself with the stock bags of IV solutions, prescription drugs, and patient supplies that I had never handled before. I didn't even know this type of pharmacy practice existed, and soon, I felt less cynical about the profession.

The pharmacists at St. Joe's rotated through the various areas of pharmacy operations, and slowly but surely, I was able to jump in and lend a hand. Of the pharmacist duties there, I most enjoyed mixing IVs and chemo drugs. I liked working with my hands and couldn't get enough of this task. I didn't enjoy entering patient orders or checking cassettes of patients' medications once the technicians had filled them. It was a mundane job that I detested, and I longed for the day when technology could take over this task so I could do something else.

In 1992, my focus was on my family and my employment as a hospital pharmacist. We had a daughter, Sarah, and our son, Raymond, would not be far behind her. We sold our house in Canfield for a nice profit and were able to pay off much of our remaining debt. I was finally able to get back some of the money and labor I had put into my brother's old house. We moved closer to Lowellville on the outskirts of the east side of Youngstown in Coitsville, and I put aside OPA and NAEP to begin enjoying life by doing what I liked to do: fixing things up.

I made the forty-five minute drive from our house in Coitsville to St. Joe's in thirty minutes when Lori went into labor with our second child, Raymond, at 3:00 a.m. I was driving a small black Mercury Tracer that Lori and I had paid a ridiculous amount for. Leasing was a new thing at the time, and while driving my previous vehicle, I was unaware that I had to stay under a certain number of miles per year. The cost for the extra 30,000 miles was carried over to the Tracer, and piece of junk or not, it got us to the hospital in time.

The first time I held Raymond in my arms, he immediately began to cry. I quickly handed him back to the nurse and noticed a small indentation in the middle of his chest from being pressed against my St. Joe's employee badge. I already had a lot of making up to do and would later wonder if his distancing himself from me was due to some deep memory of our first embrace.

Life's details, as well as precautions, are sometimes overlooked when one is busy. Lori and I bought fourteen acres of cornfield and built a house in the country. She handled the kids while I handled the hammer, and together, we finished our new home.

It was easy for me to set aside professional pharmacy issues and focus on the family that Lori and I were raising. I refrained from sending out mailings, doing interviews, and writing for publications for the three years I was at St. Joe's. I was a hospital pharmacist now, and it was certainly a different experience.

The white-coat pharmacy knowledge a hospital pharmacist uses seemed to hold greater significance than what I had experienced in a retail-chain pharmacy because it was in an urgent-care setting. Still, I remained keenly aware of the working conditions in which chain pharmacists toiled, and I understood their importance in this not-so-urgent setting. No matter how hard I tried to dismiss thoughts of the representational imbalance within the profession, a couple of drinks at a party could change all that. It was what I seemed to know best, what I had dedicated so much time and money toward, and what I felt would do the greatest good for my profession and colleagues.

Unsettled as always and finding some aspects of my job to be mundane in an ongoing soap opera of different personalities, I wanted more. I had been a pharmacist for only nine years and in 1994 I was about to give my two-weeks' notice to my fifth superior and endure the drive home to tell my wife. The four-dollar-an-hour raise I received by making the switch from hospital to independent retail pharmacy helped the resulting conversation go a bit easier.

I had made some great friends at the hospital, and I was sad to leave, but I now had three children, and the higher paycheck was calling me. Lori stayed home with our children until they were all in school, so I was now the sole breadwinner. I was already working extra hours at various independent pharmacies, in addition to my forty hours a week at St. Joe's, and this was beginning to take its toll. During this time, I set my own personal record for having worked three different pharmacies in one day. I began that day at St. Joe's, worked the afternoon at Overholt's Pharmacy in Champion, and finished the day at Kuszmaul's Pharmacy in Niles. Neither of those independent pharmacies are in business today.

I would spend the next four years of my career at Kuszmaul's learning some of the ins and outs of a mom-and-pop store. There, I saw the issues affecting this independent practice setting and put those together with what I saw while working in a chain pharmacy. The big-picture view of how the two interrelated began to stoke the fires of the NAEP again, only this time from an independent pharmacist's point of view.

The customer service we offered at Kuszmaul's was a far cry from the chain retail experience I'd had just a few short years earlier. We knew our customers' names and were given holiday baked goods in appreciation. The only issues here to stir my emotions for a lost profession were in seeing my employer's numbers decline, both in customers and in dollars reimbursed by insurance companies. These declines directly impacted my employer, who was also my friend.

Chain pharmacies were playing by different rules. They were able to dispense medications cheaply, steal our customers through exclusive contracts with the major employers in our area, and shoulder all that patient volume. From my perspective at an independent pharmacy, one pharmacist filling over three hundred prescriptions per day did not seem possible, and I reflected back on the day I'd received a call at Revco Drug from an independent pharmacist wondering how and why we were doing it. Only this time, I was the independent (employee) pharmacist asking the question.

◆ ◆ ◆

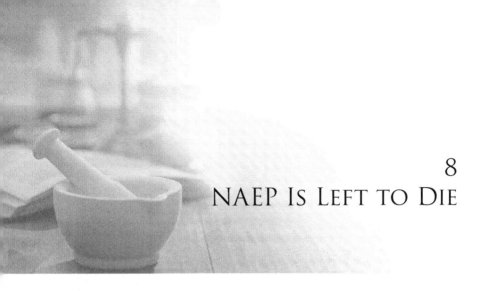

8
NAEP IS LEFT TO DIE

Secure in my job and having regained my financial footing, I started working once again on starting up the National Association of Employee Pharmacists. Although I was an employee of an independent pharmacy, not a chain, I worried that if chain pharmacists didn't speak out and rally against the working conditions they faced, they would take us all down. The profession would be severely damaged if its largest practice setting fell apart.

Independent pharmacies were disappearing, and there was talk of additional pharmacy schools opening. The demise of retail-chain pharmacy, which constitutes over 60 percent of the profession, would cause a drop in salaries as well as job opportunities. It was an issue of supply and demand in the workplace, and pharmacy wouldn't be able to handle such large numbers of unemployed pharmacists. Insurance companies were consuming our time, taking our money, and forcing customers to use mail-order pharmacy options, and chain pharmacists were along for the ride so long as their salaries continued to rise.

By the mid-1990s, the pace of activity in all areas of life was picking up. The World Wide Web was getting off the ground, and for the first time, average citizens were able to connect with one another using home computers connected to telephone land lines. We would log on and hear the modem screech while it called for an available line. If you were lucky enough to connect to the internet, it didn't necessarily mean you would stay connected, and you had to redial or unplug everything if that connection failed. We didn't seem to mind, though, because we had something we'd never had before: the ability to instantly reach a lot of people. Word processing had also come a long way by then, and different fonts and bold lettering allowed for a more professional look. I did my best to keep up with it all, knowing that these new technologies offered the connectivity I had lacked in my previous attempts to get NAEP up and running. I now had an opportunity to see whether the apathy that existed in my small region was to be found elsewhere. Welcome to the world of Windows 95!

By this point, pharmacists were openly complaining about the high volume they were expected to handle, and national publications were reporting increases in dispensing errors. Computers could also now gather data on hospital admissions related to medication misuse, and the numbers were not good. OBRA-90 and Drug Use Review laws were on the books, and yet, there seemed to be no change in our dispensing practices. In fact, things only seemed to be getting worse. It was still several years before our nation's opioid epidemic would catch widespread public attention, but computer data was providing hints that something was on the horizon.

In 1996, Purdue Pharmaceuticals marketed OxyContin in 10, 20, 40, and 80 milligram strengths, while also claiming that the adverse reaction known as "addiction" was not a concern. That year Purdue realized sales of $48 million. If chain pharmacists had been willing to speak out against a pace that kept them from document-ing adverse reactions and engaged in professional associations to pressure corporate thinkers into aligning themselves with lawful practice, Purdue's false claims would have been uncovered soon. Instead, years of professional silence provided all the cover this manufacturer needed to market a 160 milligram tablet, and Purdue's sales soared to $1.1 billion by the year 2000. But in 1996, the same year addiction numbers began to rise, professional apathy still kept pharmacists silent. Just as concerning, the drug use review boards that each state was to have in place to catch trends of abuse and overuse were equally silent.

We all talked among ourselves about the crazy days we had behind our pharmacy counters and laughed about our crazy customer inter-actions. Workplace conditions were deteriorating at the slow pace that often escapes recognition, but it was happening none the less. And most pharmacists felt it happening.

I had yet to put two and two—OBRA-90 laws and their viola-tions—together, so I wasn't addressing this as I once again tried to fire up NAEP. I was still focused on the fact that chain pharmacy was huge and was the only practice setting that didn't have a democratic representative organization of its own. The fact that pharmacists in this largest of settings had no means of comfortably speaking their piece was my only concern, and although I recognized that nothing good would come of this void, I didn't yet understand that there were real legal violations occurring. Why would I? I was fill-ing prescriptions just as fast and in the same manner as everyone else, and no one from the Ohio Board of Pharmacy objected. I knew about OBRA-90, but like everyone else, I didn't have time to step back from the grind of work to implement it. There was no professional association pressuring us to recognize and abide by it. The law was passed in 1990, and states were given three years to comply. Perhaps if that time frame had been shortener, the profession and its players might have felt more urgency to put the law into practice.

With my new home computer and all its futuristic capabilities, I began to organize NAEP, feeling confident that my timing was right. A new, higher level of workplace misery was beginning to emerge, and we all talked about it. All indications were that the time was right for these chain pharmacists to join such an organization, speak out about their unprofessional working conditions, and do so in the safety of numbers.

I wrote my one and only NAEP newsletter, Volume 1, Number 1, after months of phone calls that led me to believe that if I could use the computer to reach the masses, those masses would be comforted knowing that they weren't alone. It was my best attempt to convey that there was safety in numbers, and if chain pharmacists had even a tinge of civic responsibility, understood the conditions they were working in, and appreciated the democratic country they lived in, my effects might be received positively.

I have but one original copy of the newsletter. I was thirty-four years old when I wrote these words in 1996; mailed them to pharmacists, associations, and publications; and put them out on the World Wide Web. Please see **Addendum 3** for the full version, but here are the important points I was trying to make:

NATIONAL ASSOCIATION OF EMPLOYEE PHARMACISTS
The Voice of the Employee/Chain Pharmacist Volume 1, Number 1 1996
Can The Majority Afford to Remain Silent?

> *The current state of pharmacy might lead one to believe that some-one's interests are not being protected. The PEW report estimates a surplus of 40,000 pharmacists by the year 2000 and has recommended reducing the number of pharmacy schools by 25% by the*

year 2005. The public is mandating (OBRA-90) action to serve us with notice of their discontent at the high cost of medication misuse. Our professional environment grows busier and more confusing in the wake of higher volume, lower margins, and 3rd Party management. Even more sad is the report that we have the second-highest risk of suicide among more than 250 occupations analyzed by NIOSH.

We are a concerned group of Employee/Chain pharmacists asking you to consider what we believe is an important pharmacy issue. **We are the National Association of Employee Pharmacists (NAEP)**, and we believe that a professional organization to directly represent the interests of pharmacy's largest practice setting is long overdue.

Oh No! Not Another Association!

We have national associations that represent Hospital, Independent, Clinical, Consulting, and Scientific pharmacists. We also have associations that represent pharmacy educators, pharmacy lawyers, pharmacy boards, pharmaceutical manufacturers, pharmaceutical distributors, owners of pharmacy chains, managed care pharmacy, and many more. Those who benefit from joining their own practice setting association can likewise join the professional organizations available to all. The 50 state associations represent all pharmacists within given boundaries and AphA represents all pharmacists within the 50 states. So, how has it come to pass that amid so many organizations representing so many other interests that the Employee, who constitutes the majority, has been without such benefits?

IMPORTANT UPDATE:
NAEP WASTES NO TIME REPRESENTING YOU:

The American Pharmaceutical Association invited Ray Carlson, R.Ph. (NAEP-Ohio) to discuss Employee/Chain quality of work-life and professional representation issues at the August 24th AphA-APPM Executive Committee and Section Chairs meeting in Washington D.C. A motion was passed to establish a task force to assess Employee/Chain work-life conditions, seek standardization of 3rd party plans, and recommend name and/or structural changes to AphA sections to provide for better representation.

AphA is our association to protect all of pharmacy. As NAEP is to one setting, so too is AphA to all. We have opened the door enough to see that together we must turn the tide for our setting and the profession. NAEP will have a seat on this task force, and we will need and welcome your ideas and input. Please, make the time to respond.

There was no response to this mailing, and although two national pharmacy publications briefly mentioned it in one of their monthly issues, NAEP was apparently not as grand an idea as I thought. Months of pressuring chain pharmacists to recognize how they could create change had turned into years, and I was once again disappointed by their lack of interest. Still, I'd said what I wanted to say, and twenty-five years later, I would feel some sense of dark vindication knowing that these words were written well in advance of the suffering that was to come.

Instant Messenger, real-time chatting, and the ability to filter profiles to focus on a targeted audience was now possible, and I spent a fair amount of time spreading the love for NAEP. I soon found that I liked "snail mail" better than the World Wide Web; at least an empty P.O. box wouldn't contain the condescending comments that came in an instant when opening messages on a computer. I fought an uphill battle every time I entered a chat group. When one chain pharmacist accused me of being some sort of "Jesus," I shut off my computer and put it away. I would never again debate the need for an NAEP to pharmacists I did not know on the web. I was just an ordinary guy trying to warn chain pharmacists of what was in store for them, and it was unfortunate for me that I was twenty-five years too early for them to listen. Their situation had deteriorated to such an extent that any suggestion that a professional association could help them was met with laughter and cynicism.

I spent a considerable amount of time, money, and energy on this mission over the years, and I felt as though I had delivered my message as clearly as I could and to as many as I could. My sample size was large, and my methods were about as direct as they could possibly be. Chain pharmacists were going to do what they were going to do, and nothing I—or OPA or APhA—said could move them to join as one and speak out. I was again facing the effects of professional apathy.

Not long after my trip to D.C. to address the American Pharmaceutical Association, my organization folded a second time; this time, for good. I had wasted nearly six years and endured one frustration after another when I could have been enjoying tipsy conversations about sports or politics instead of pharmacy democracy. The apathy among chain pharmacists was a national phenomenon, and my web mailings, direct mailings, and litany of phone conversations were enough to show me this.

Perhaps I should have played on pharmacists' sympathies by mentioning that I addressed the APhA committee after having broken my neck just weeks earlier. I wore a neck brace while delivering my presentation with the help of an overhead projector. I was searching for any angle I could use to reach the chain pharmacist, so I'm not sure why I didn't mention my own personal suffering on their behalf. I wish I had been able to enjoy the time I spent in that beautiful APhA building without the discomfort of this medical device, but I also feel fortunate for being one of the lucky few who sustains such a break and is still able to stand upright.

The accident occurred while we were on vacation with friends in Ocean City, hoping to enjoy some time away with our three young children. We had enjoyed a day or so at the beach when my mind wandered away from family and toward the important NAEP presentation I had been asked to give to our nation's top pharmacy association. I pulled a nearly all-nighter on the balcony of our condo writing my presentation. The next day, with senses dulled and reflexes tired, I raced my son on a boogie board and lost. A rogue wave managed to get under my board and drive my head into the ocean's sandy bottom with enough force for me to hear the break. I instantly felt the pain. I crawled back to my beach towel and rested for a moment before denying to my wife that anything was wrong. I resolved to go back to the condo to sit in the hot tub and maybe find some relief with ibuprofen, but after nearly passing out when I stood up, I realized that no amount of over-the-counter anti-inflammatory was going to fix what was clearly broken.

No one, including myself, would have guessed that I had just broken my neck, so we walked to the car and drove to the nearest emergency clinic. Sitting in the waiting room was unbearable, as was the walk to the examination room. The next thing I knew, I was on a helicopter heading to Baltimore's Shock Trauma Hospital. Lori made the frantic three-hour drive while our friends watched our children, and after only one fender bender, she arrived safely at my side.

I was very fortunate that the break was a clean compression fracture of C2 and C3 and that no discs were out of place. That was huge! It was a quick heal of just a few months, but not before enduring weeks of pain the likes of which I had never experienced before. It was so intense that I was nauseated. This accident and the resulting pain would forever change my opinion about responsible use of opioids by those patients who were truly in need of pain relief. My father-in-law had to endure the ride home from Maryland with someone who had nothing on his mind but pharmacy democracy and NAEP.

After my presentation, the APhA staff took me out to dinner, and I had a drink or two. My brace had become uncomfortable after weeks of constantly wearing it, and the alcohol seemed to relax my neck muscles enough for me to remove it when I got back to the hotel. I took it off that night and never wore it again. APhA's generosity seemed to heal me in more ways than one.

I had an adrenaline rush when I first met John Gans, PharmD., and Tom Menighan, B.S. Pharm., MBA, inside the walls of APhA's beautiful, grand building in Washington, D.C., on Constitution Avenue directly across the street from the Lincoln Memorial. It's probably why the memory has stuck with me. To this day, I can precisely picture the offices where we first spoke, the beautiful rotunda where I signed in, and the stunning framed portraits on the walls. I was honored to have some of their time, and I enjoyed our conversations inside such a beautiful structure in our nation's capital. I took a picture of the front of the building on my way out and have it hanging on my wall behind my bar in the basement.

I was young at the time, and I wonder what they thought of someone attempting to organize a national professional association of chain pharmacists. The idea was as grand as the building we stood inside, but my conversations with John and Tom led me to believe that it wasn't as novel as I'd previously thought. Both had tried one form of representation after another over the years, and all of them had failed. Apparently, the chain pharmacist was unapproachable and unmoving where democracy was concerned.

The number of chain pharmacists who Join APhA is pathetic. If only half the chain pharmacists joined, the organization's membership would quadruple. There has long been a debate about the reasons behind chain pharmacists' apathy, and perhaps what has now befallen them is somewhat deserved. Both John Gans and Tom Menighan recognized that chain pharmacists were absent from pharmacy discussions, and they would collectively serve three decades as CEO of APhA without having found a way to move this group to action. Tom himself was a chain pharmacist for five years prior to his involvement in professional organizations and, as such, was intimately aware of the challenges faced by this group.

In the end, I realized what others had already realized. APhA was happy to give each of our NAEP members—about 125 of them in total—one free year of membership, and I bowed out gracefully. I doubt that even with all the technology now available, I would be able to move this group to associate with one another. No real-time video message or meme or hashtag is going to overcome apathy. Chain pharmacists cannot envision an escape because they are blind to the benefits of a professional organization, and this is probably why they're still without an organization to call their own.

Chain pharmacists could completely take over APhA, our national organization for all pharmacists, and with their staggering numbers, dominate offices and committees and pass any sort of resolution they wanted. But beaten down professionally and propped up by cash, they think too little of themselves and the profession to want to expend any further energy on pharmacy-related issues once they exit their stores that are owned by others. The chain pharmacist community had sealed its own professional fate by not coming together to speak out about their working conditions, and the public would pay the price when the debt that was created by their silence needed to be paid.

Now that I had put away NAEP for good, I felt as though I needed to make a change in my life. I needed to retreat into a different part of the woods, hoping to not leave tracks that would tell others of the embarrassing places I had been. All the travel, time, and money I spent on this effort over the years had been wasted, and I needed to put it out of my mind and move on.

◆ ◆ ◆

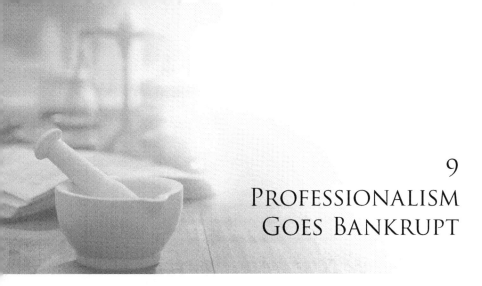

9
PROFESSIONALISM
GOES BANKRUPT

On my last day of work at Kuszmaul's Pharmacy, the owner, Gary Kuszmaul, walked in with a six-pack of beer at closing, and we sat on the floor in the back room and talked. He told me about the day his pharmacy was robbed by a guy in a long coat that he used to hide a shotgun as he entered the pharmacy. He pulled it out when he was halfway up the main aisle as he approached the back pharmacy counter. The guy ordered everyone to get on the floor in the back, he grabbed what he wanted, and out the door he went. He was later arrested, served his time, and came back to the store to apologize. I don't think Gary was ever the same after that, and he admitted as much on that last day we shared together in his pharmacy. His store was later sold for a fraction of what it might have been valued at just a few years earlier, and a restaurant moved in to serve the public's interest.

By now, my NAEP reputation had cooled, and my rebel ways were never mentioned in job interviews. I accepted my seventh job with the retail chain Phar-Mor, who had just opened a new store five minutes from my house in Poland, Ohio. I no longer had to make the thirty-five-minute drive to Niles and would enjoy more weekends and holidays off. Since it was a new store with competition on every corner, the prescription volume would be low for probably the first couple of years. It wouldn't be a breakneck pace, and I could handle that. I didn't have an "every man for himself" attitude, but our children were keeping us busy, and I wanted to spend more time with them. I packed up my NAEP propaganda in a box, where it would sit for the next twenty years. I was moving on to raise a family.

Many of my friends, including my brother-in-law, Mike, worked for Phar-Mor. I was allowed to display my antique prescription bottles in my new store, and I received an employee discount on merchandise. Best of all, I was receiving seven dollars an hour more than I had at Kuszmaul's, and I didn't have to shovel snow or change ballasts in the ceiling lights. Salaries were going nowhere but up at the end of the century. I was becoming financially stable thanks to free-market forces.

I existed at Phar-Mor, blessed that my store was a slow one, but I didn't like it. Corporate distractions were beginning to take on new meanings, and visits from supervisors were no longer exchanges of mutual respect or even friendliness. We all saw how corporate treated out-front managers, and it broke my heart. Often, these managers were men with small children to provide for, and the hours they worked for the money they were paid made interacting with them awkward. At the time of my hiring, Phar-Mor had just emerged from one bankruptcy and was teetering on the verge of another. Perhaps this is why supervisors had such an aggressive attitude toward staff.

When my supervisor emailed me to inform me that I was about to receive a raise, I asked that it be distributed evenly among my pharmacy technicians and out-front manager instead. Although the extra money would have been helpful, corporate pharmacy leaves a professional void as well as a personal one, and I hoped that I might be able to exchange this pay raise for a feeling of fellow humanity with my coworkers. Many chain pharmacists I knew and talked to would gladly have done the same.

There was an ever-present disparity that I couldn't escape, knowing that those who were working just as hard as I was and receiving the same amount, if not more, customer abuse, were being paid about a fifth of what I was as a pharmacist. My attempt to ease this disparity between those who were carrying as much customer and insurance weight as I was rejected. I was simply informed that "my request was not possible."

There were many busy chain pharmacies in our area at the time. CVS and Phar-Mor seemed to have the most pharmacists complaining about their prescription volume. I knew a lot of pharmacists and was as good a barometer of "busy" as any, and any of them who claimed they didn't feel the pressure never looked in the mirror to see the bags under their eyes or the varicose veins under their pants. The stories we shared were as professionally mind-boggling then as they are today; only now, they're shared on social media. We knew which chain pharmacies dominated the market in our area, and I personally marveled at those pharmacists who woke up every morning with the financial drive to work at them.

Over the years, I worked at most of the Phar-Mors in my area, and they all shared the same lust for volume. Despite the numbers, it was possible to observe the same dispensing patterns at each. My career would eventually have me working behind the counter at almost all the CVS and Giant Eagle stores in two counties, so I have firsthand knowledge of what pharmacists were experiencing; it was the same professional cesspool everywhere. The entire industry in at least these two counties had tossed aside pharmacists' responsibilities and slowly but surely buried them in corporate distractions and sales gimmicks.

I found that it was the female pharmacists who strove to uphold some level of professionalism and maintain some semblance of lawful conduct, and you could see the stress in their faces. They were better on their best days than the male pharmacists could ever hope to be, and worse than males on their worst days when timing demanded it and nothing seemed to matter, since volume made it impossible to be your best. The pace was such that a twelve-hour day flew by in agony, letters on the screen blurred with warnings and overrides, and deep down inside, we all knew that we had not been educated to perform this way. Unfortunately for all, we didn't have the time to consider the illegal nature of it all.

We didn't have the time to phone doctors or talk to patients about concerns we might have about the prescriptions we were filling. We spent far more time on the phone talking to insurance companies than entering notes in a patient's profile. Techs were given override codes when a warning flashed across the screen, and drugs were handed out a window with a smile and some catchy phrase the company wanted us to say that was every bit as ridiculous as those we used when answering the phone.

Book-cooking had forced the Phar-Mor chain into bankruptcy in 1992. The company was founded by Mickey Monus and David Shapira in 1982, and its corporate headquarters were in downtown Youngstown. David Shapira, who is now the executive chairman of Giant Eagle, claimed to have no knowledge of Phar-Mor's book-cooking scheme. After Monus was sent to prison for his role in the billion-dollar fraud, half of the once grand Phar-Mor stores were closed or sold, and the company emerged from bankruptcy in 1995 only to find itself having to go head-to-head against other major retailers like Walmart, which were entering the pharmacy space. Corporate leaders with a mindset based in deceit fashioned pharmacy business models that involved leveraging their ability to "power buy" and make up their lost margin by focusing on volume.

Phar-Mor was forced into bankruptcy again in 2001, and even though we could all see the writing on the wall, we were told that everything would be okay. In 2002, a judge approved the sale of the company, and Phar-Mor was liquidated—but not before it displayed one last astounding measure of unprofessionalism.

The way the Phar-Mor stores closed was a testimony to the apathy of those pharmacists who ran the various prescription departments and their blind obedience to orders that placed patient safety at risk. It turns out that the value of a pharmacy is determined by the number of patient records on file and active prescriptions filled. A potential buyer would look at the number of customers and active prescriptions they were handling and pay accordingly. If the company selling a pharmacy could entice patients to transfer their prescriptions to their store, the added value when the sale went through would be greater than the loss they would incur in enticing new patients.

At a managers' meeting near Pittsburgh, we were deceived into believing that the company was going to do everything in its power to emerge from bankruptcy and continue operations. As I listened, I reflected that others might feel good about this pep talk, keep their chins up, and fight the good fight, but not me. I wasn't fooled.

Shortly after our manager's meeting, Phar-Mor advertised "$25 of free in-store merchandise for every prescription transferred." The free-for-all had begun. Customers were looking for any pill bottles from other pharmacies they could find and handed them to us in exchange for twenty-five-dollars-worth of stuff: old bottles, new bottles, outdated bottles, dangerous-if-taken-again bottles. We saw it all. I had one "new" customer bring in sixteen prescription bottles from various other pharmacies. They received their refills, filled a cart with four-hundred-dollars-worth of Phar-Mor merchandise, and out the door they went. My professional services were being used to inflate the value of a store through the illusion of customer relationships that did not exist. I was convinced that the end was near.

The depth to which OBRA-90 had been violated, and allowed to do so without any organized protest, had found a new bottom of deceit. The distraction caused by having to call other pharmacies to transfer "new patient" prescriptions allowed who knows how many illegitimate prescriptions to pass through our pharmacy counters. A legitimate medical purpose for old and unnecessary prescription vials found with dust on them when taken from medicine cabinets became a way to pad volume in a deceptively legitimate way. Who knows how many physicians were able to prescribe drugs during that time when our ability to scrutinize them had been compromised by the chaos created by our employers?

Buried in this pace of free antibiotics and diabetic medications, calling insurance companies, and having to learn yet another new computer or fax system were the opioids that passed through our hurried process. The same handful of scumbag doctors in the area who would eventually lose their licenses were making a killing off the worker's compensation and Medicaid patients that they demanded to see every thirty days. They never put refills on the prescriptions that were allowed to have refills, and the Schedule II narcotics that could not be refilled were included in the pile of prescriptions each month. We spent much more time typing in the same monthly prescriptions as if they were new than we would if these physicians had simply authorized a refill. We knew what they were doing: they wanted to bill the patients for a monthly office visit.

Did we have time to notice whether someone looked like they were abusing an opioid? Was the patient who didn't have the normal look of someone taking OxyContin three times a day actually selling their pills? Did we note our concerns or suspicions in the computer so the Board of Pharmacy could investigate? Did the Board of Pharmacy ever look at patient profiles to see if we were concerned about an addiction or diversion problem? Simply put, no. Chain pharmacists had no time because of the number of independent pharmacies they had put out of business. The Board of Pharmacy had no time because they were too focused on the problems that resulted from this volume. Medication errors must have been higher than anyone thought—but not with Schedule II narcotics, because they had to be typed in anew with each fill, and they always received "extra care." That level of care should have included looking out for misuse and abuse, but in practice, it didn't. Corporate chain pharmacy, and all their little games like the $25 coupon incentive, buried their works so completely that no one dare mentioned adding the task of OBRA-90 compliance.

Chain pharmacists weren't expected to be policemen, but we were supposed to convert our suspicions into patient profile notes, especially if we thought someone was abusing a drug. That way, the Board of Pharmacy would have documentation if they were investigating a particular doctor or patient. Our duty was not to engage in face-to-face confrontations with abusers, but to provide a paper trail for agencies and the police to follow. There was too great a risk to pharmacists personally to get in the face of someone who had little to lose.

I confronted such a patient just once while working at Phar-Mor, and I soon regretted it. It involved an early refill of Xanax, which I refused to fill. The patient called me later that evening, threatening me, and sure enough, when I went out to my car that night, the head-lights of a vehicle were aimed directly at me in the otherwise-empty parking lot. This continued for the next several evenings. In the end, I had to be escorted out of the building by a police officer every night for two weeks. My home was just down the road from the store, and my children were small at the time. I resolved to never again risk my safety or theirs by confronting an abuser. Our role is to provide help to future investigations by communicating our suspicions to the Board, and if the Board has a wealth of patient entries to go on, making an arrest and stopping the abuse is that much easier for them.

In 2001, knowing that I was leaving Pharm-Mor soon and feeling the frustrations of corporate pharmacy, I allowed myself to have a rare but precious verbal altercation with a patient. This patient called me at the store after returning home with a prescription I had filled for her. She'd had a lengthy bout of diarrhea, and her physician prescribed a common medication to treat it called metronidazole. After I said hello, she immediately began complaining about her insurance copay and demanded to know why I hadn't run her prescription through under her husband's card. I explained that I didn't see that insurance in the computer and that she hadn't offered us his card. Then, I threw caution to the wind and began to scold her about her attitude—and everyone else's—when having prescriptions filled. I detailed just how important and dangerous this medication was, how dangerous her condition could be if not treated correctly, and everything I was supposed to do to help her if I could only get away from these damn insurance questions. She didn't care about the professional services I could offer her or how I could help her with her condition and keep her safe from harm. The chain pharmacy I worked for—and all the other chain pharmacies in town—didn't care, either. But I had successfully gotten off my chest what I and many other pharmacists longed to say, and I was able to do so because I was leaving. The other pharmacists working for Phar-Mor had to stay and battle all the distractions that corporate America had put in their way.

I found another job, put in my two-weeks' notice, and encouraged other Phar-Mor pharmacist to do the same. I knew the company wasn't telling the truth about not going under, and I wasn't about to stick around to find out when it would happen.

Not long thereafter, Phar-Mor's front doors were chained shut. A sign informed customers that all prescriptions had been transferred and could now be filled at the local Giant Eagle. A CEO within Phar-Mor was also a CEO within Giant Eagle, and no one seemed to care that prescription files had been artificially padded for the sale. The business model of deceit and danger merely crossed the street. I got out just in time while others scrambled for the limited openings to be found. I was about to begin work as a pharmacist in another practice setting that was unfamiliar to me: home care.

◆ ◆ ◆

10
LEARNING THE BUSINESS OF STERILE COMPOUNDING

As I exited my beat up Mercury Tracer, walked across the parking lot, and entered the lobby of MVI HomeCare, I thought to myself that I knew nothing about what a home-infusion pharmacist even did, and with that, I had no idea how I was going to make it through the interview. I was about to meet the owners of this home-infusion company, Dale Damoli, R.Ph., and his partner, Kevin McGuire, and I was sure I'd bomb it. I was clueless about home IV therapy and dosing of antibiotics and Total Parenteral Nutritions (TPNs) and I had never prepared a narcotic pain pump for a hospice patient. Worse yet, I had no reasonable explanation for why I'd held so many different pharmacy jobs at such a young age.

However, my answers must have been what Dale and Kevin wanted to hear because they offered me the job, and I accepted it. I gave my two-weeks' notice at Phar-Mor, accepted the pay cut, and hoped to find some humanity in this type of pharmacy. Dale and Kevin were the founders and sole owners of the company, which meant there was no corporate food chain to contend with. It was a family-run business of decent size and stability, the employees apparently enjoyed their jobs, and the role of the pharmacist was much more clinical than what I had experienced before. I could tell from researching the position that I had a lot to learn if I was going to survive in this world, and there could be no mistakes in this critically clinical pharmacy position.

I lucked out with Mariellen Warvel, R.Ph., as my mentor. She taught me everything I needed to know. I had experience preparing IVs, thanks to my time at St. Joe's, but now I would be dosing TPNs, calculating antibiotic drip rates, and preparing pain management cassettes for hospice patients. Mariellen was both professional and funny, and she had me up and running in this field in no time. Just a few months after I started, Mariellen had to take a leave of absence, putting me in charge of all pharmacy operations. In less than a year, I had transitioned from a pharmacist working for a big retail chain whose only worry was running out of twenty-five-dollar coupons to a pharmacist reading lab values and calculating TPNs. I was clinically and professionally free from bondage.

At the time of my hiring, MVI HomeCare was located in an old motel that was split up into many different sections while they were putting the finishing touches on a brand-new building. In a matter of weeks, we were packing drugs and equipment for the move into our new space. The new facility gave me my first look at a true anteroom and cleanroom. These are sterile air-filled rooms in which IV hoods are placed and IV solutions are mixed.

Home-infusion pharmacy requires a pharmacist to be on call 24/7. Nurses cared for patients in their homes, and when drugs or supplies were missing from an order, new orders came from hospital discharges, or patient lab results necessitated a change in drug dosages, our pagers went off, and we had to run into the office to take care of whatever was needed. Cell phones weren't commonplace back then, so we used pagers, which just sent us a number to call for instructions.

This position required putting a lot of miles on my vehicle. Sometimes, after mixing a few bags of IV drugs and gathering supplies, I would meet a nurse at a drop-off point or take it directly to a patient's house. I was paid whenever I had to drive into the office, and I received a few dollars an hour for those times when all was quiet, but I still struggled with having to leave my children's concerts, ball games, and family gatherings only to say that I would be back as soon as I could.

Still, it was a nine-to-five job and nothing like the twelve-hour days of retail pharmacy, and I felt good about the pharmacy services I provided. I was paid two dollars an hour for the time I was on call and received regular wages if I had to prepare and order. I enjoyed my time there and felt respected for the pharmacy duties I performed. I calculated the amounts of vitamins needed in a TPN, dosed Vancomycin according to lab results, sucked every drop out of a vial of morphine, and answered the phone without worry or concern. I also enjoyed working with everyone at MVI. There were no personality conflicts with any of the nurses or staff, and my friendships with those who worked in the pharmacy soon grew into a brotherhood of sorts.

One could easily imagine that I would stay there forever. Unfortunately, a perfect storm brewed—mild though it was—that combined a gripe of mine with the job recruiting efforts of MVI's competitor. And it all came together after an incident with a nurse.

One evening, around midnight, a nurse who was caring for a hospice patient paged me. I rarely expressed frustration about late-night pages, especially regarding hospice patients, and the situation wasn't all that upsetting, but the nurse apparently misinterpreted my words. The next day, I was called into Kevin's office for the way I had spoken to her. It wasn't a scolding—more like a reminder to be understanding—but this was one of the rare times when I was summoned to the offices down the hall for any reason. I had good ideas to share, ideas that had already saved money and improved care quality, yet it was rare for me to be asked to attend meetings, let alone to discuss operations with the owners. Timing and bitterness met up with a job offer, and despite MVI's offer to increase my pay if I stayed, I gave my two-week notice for the ninth time, and I had to explain to Lori yet again why I couldn't seem to build up my 401K.

In 2002, I began working for HM Home Pharmacy, the home infusion branch of Humility of Mary Health Systems and St. Elizabeth's Hospital in Youngstown. Although the home care portion of the hospital system was off campus, we were part of the largest hospital system in the Youngstown area. I was the supervisor of HM Home Pharmacy and was part of HM Home Care, which was supervised by my superior, Rod Carnifax.

I already knew that large hospitals came with layers of administration, and being the head of a department, I wasn't going to have to worry about not being called into meetings. Since my time at MVI had prepared me to assume the role of pharmacy director with very little training, I was able to hit the ground running with eyes wide open to what was happening around me. The tunnel vision that sometimes accompanies new positions and new tasks was absent for the first time in a long time.

The HM Home Pharmacy department was in the basement of a not-so-nice building, there was no cleanroom, and there seemed to be no sterile procedures for mixing IVs. A new building design was in the hands of an architect who had prepared basic plans to which I would be able to add walls and determine room sizes and the location of equipment. My superior, Rod, seemed to rely heavily on my input. He was the consummate manager in charge, big and strong, with an energetic and encouraging personality. He was fair and just, expected accountability, and encouraged participation and teamwork.

The time I spent at HM Home Pharmacy was vital for the business (RC Compounding Services, LLC) that I would start from the ground up, and it would happen because of a single prescription that was faxed to my department in error. The fax was a prescription order that was supposed to go to a compounding pharmacy in Florida, where it would be filled and then shipped back to St. Elizabeth's Hospital. I called St. Elizabeth's pharmacy department and asked what I was supposed to do with the fax; I was told to shred it, as it had been sent in error. Looking at it, I asked myself why we weren't able to prepare it here. It was an order for morphine prepared from raw powder, diluted, sterilized, and then dispensed in a syringe for use by a physician to fill a pain pump. I asked Rod the same question, and he gave me the green light to investigate it.

If regulations governing the compounding of intrathecal syringes containing drug meant for injection into the spine were what they are today, we would never have been able to mix these types of drugs. At the time, though, the joke was that if you had a barrier hood, you could mix sterile drugs in the parking lot. A barrier hood is a glass box that circulates very clean air. It's accessed by sticking your arms into heavy rubber gloves while mixing the sterile drugs. It prevents bacteria from entering the final drug solution that is administered to the patient. This is of particular importance when that final solution will be injected into the intrathecal space of the spine that has little or no immune system to protect it.

My wife's cousin, Joe Flora, happened to be the head of purchasing at St. Elizabeth's, and he found a barrier hood in the bowels of the hospital basement. Miraculously, it had never been used. He called me to tell me that he'd located what he thought I was looking for and that he was going to have it shipped to our home infusion department ten miles away. If that phone call had instead been to tell me that he couldn't locate one, we wouldn't have started our sterile prescription service, and I probably wouldn't be writing this story. Instead, Joe delivered on his promise, and I spent the next several weeks learning the art of mixing sterile drugs from what we called "bulk powders"—in essence, turning a dirty drug into a clean one. It was a service that few in the state of Ohio were providing because it was risky to prepare a sterile drug from non-sterile drug powder that was to be injected into the spine, and I was about to learn it for myself. And all because someone had pressed the wrong button.

The difference between the types of injectable drugs we had been mixing and this new type I was about to learn was that this new dosage form had an ingredient that was considered "dirty." The bulk drug that was to be mixed, in this case it was morphine, was a white powder that was not sterile. It needed to be weighed out on a scale, mixed with an IV solution, and then sterilized by either running the solution through a very fine filter that would trap the bacteria, or placed in an oven for an hour or two and heated. Most hospitals, clinics, and compounding pharmacies simply mix a drug that is already sterile with a solution that is already sterile, and since both components being mixed were drugs and solutions obtained from an FDA inspected manufacturer, the risk of bacterial contamination is minimized.

Under normal circumstances, it would not be necessary to compound drug dosages from raw drug powder were it not for the special mix of different drugs physicians wanted, or specific doses required that were not already commercially available by a manufacturer. More important was the bottlenecked supply chain of drugs that caused many to be out of stock. Sometimes there was no commercially available drug for months at a time, and patients would have to go without were it not for the ability of compounding pharmacies to make dosages from scratch. We were a manufacturer of sorts, coming to the rescue of a fragile drug supply chain.

I took the time to research the relevant literature, compile sterile procedures, and begin offering this service of providing sterile intrathecal syringes just in time for us to break ground on our department's new home. I oversaw the construction from start to finish and ordered all the equipment necessary to provide a safe, sterile compounding area. My office was nice and big, with two full walls of shelving that displayed many of my antique prescription bottles.

Rod held our weekly "Ops" meeting in the conference room, and I had the opportunity to speak at each one. He went around the room, and everyone spoke whether they had something prepared or not. In essence, I was sitting in on Business Management 101 each week. At the time, I had no idea how valuable these leadership lessons would be or the extent to which I would incorporate them into my own business.

One difference between retail pharmacy and institutional pharmacy is the limited number of people you'll interact with every day in institutional pharmacy. I first recognized this while working at St. Joe's, and it admittedly played a role in my decision to leave. Every now and then, my work life felt like a never-ending soap opera, and although close friendships are nice when things are going well, when friendships turn sour, the days drag in misery. I didn't have this in retail. Each day, I interacted with over a hundred different personalities from all walks of life, and everyone had a different story to tell. Unfortunately, the tragedy of personality clashes would play out at

HM Home Pharmacy as it had nowhere else I'd worked. It eventually became more than I wanted to deal with.

I felt that I had learned all I needed to learn and that the time had come for me to satisfy my inner entrepreneur. In the short time I had the reins of HM Home Pharmacy I had increased business eight-fold, and just as I once thought my pharmacy customers would follow me from Struthers to Lowellville, I was convinced that those doctors who liked dealing with me would follow me no matter where I went. It was a bold and somewhat conceited attitude to take, but the products and services they were using were ones I had thought up, and I knew I hadn't exhausted my ideas. I had a good work ethic, my ideas made money for someone else, and I wanted to be my own boss and decide for myself who I would work with. I was going to start my own sterile compounding business.

The idea of starting my own business from nothing was easy for me to sell to myself, but convincing my wife would be a whole other conversation. I decided to run the idea past my father first. We were sitting on lawn chairs in the garage of my sister's house, celebrating my parents' fiftieth wedding anniversary in 2006, when I explained my business model to him. I wanted to open my own sterile compounding pharmacy, and I felt good about my prospects of being able to obtain enough customers to make a go of it. My dad gave me the thumbs-up, and with that backing, I decided to run the idea past Lori and see where it got me.

By now, Lori was back at work, but we were still somewhat living paycheck to paycheck, and it was a bit of an argument when I first told her about my idea. I had no business plan, no money, and no customers yet, so I understood her frustration when her nervous tone elevated. This would be my tenth job change, and I was only forty-four years old. I had yet to stay with any employer long enough to be vested in any retirement plan. Her father sat me down to discuss this decision

I was about to make. He wanted to play devil's advocate to be sure that I had thought things through. I always respected his opinions, and after our talk, I felt good about moving forward with my idea. Lori allowed me to quit HM only when I had secured another full-time job, and with that, I was ready to give my notice.

It did not seem right for me to continue to work at HM Home Pharmacy while starting my business that would compete with it, so I told Rod that I wanted to take some time off to write a book. I shouldn't have given this reason with such passivity, given how difficult I now find the task of writing to be, but it was something I'd always hoped to do one day, and it seemed like a good enough reason at the time.

It was 2006 and pharmacy jobs were still somewhat plentiful. I had not been involved in any controversial association work that would scare off a retail pharmacy recruiter, so I felt good about my prospects of finding another full-time job. My wife was satisfied with that, and I began to make phone calls and complete applications to return once again to the life of a retail chain pharmacist. I had been absent from that practice setting for nearly six years and had no idea what to expect if I landed a job there. Everything would be different this time around . . . I had it in my mind to be my own boss preparing sterile intrathecal syringes from raw drug powder. I was going to return to the chain retail setting that I hated so much to cover my bills at home while starting my own business.

I believed in myself and I was more than ready to begin thinking about what I would call my business. My frequent job changes were akin to changing classrooms in a real-world school of pharmacy. I soaked up as much knowledge as I could from each job I had, and now it was my time to take my degree and help others as I thought best. I would create my own pension plan.

❖ ❖ ❖

11
The Best and Worst Professional Experience of My Life

Shortly after I began my search for a job that would tide me over financially, I got one with the retail chain CVS, and I immediately gave my two weeks' notice to HM Home Pharmacy. I packed up my antique bottles, cleaned out my office, and headed out to begin yet again at a retail chain pharmacy that was fifty minutes from my house in another county. Although I was on the lookout for the workplace ugliness that others had warned about, I was in training and was being pampered for the first couple of weeks, and all seemed to be going okay. Everyone was cordial, the training material had pretty pictures of happy customers, and I was watching videos filled with happy faces and happy places. Hmm, maybe things aren't so bad in chain retail after all?

I was shown a world of fluffy puppies and unicorns by CVS when I started, and it was enough for my wife and me to have conversations about my ability work there instead of taking the risk of opening my own compounding pharmacy. We both had cold feet. We had just gotten out of debt and were doing okay; working for CVS was a pay increase; and my training with the company was going well. With memories of my failed Carlson's Riverside Pharmacy forcing me to question my decision to open my own business, I was riding a teeter-totter in considering what was best for my family. Should I pursue my own business and risk near-bankruptcy again? Maybe I should just stay at CVS and enjoy the higher pay.

My complacency at CVS would end, however, when I began working alone behind the pharmacy counter with limited technician staff to help me. The thought that I could just hang there for the next twenty-five years until my retirement dissipated quickly.

It was a busy day of new and refill prescriptions at CVS when I made my decision. The phones and drive-thru window were constant distractions. Our stock of narcotics was sitting in a tote on the floor, waiting to be put away. There was no way that the number of people behind the pharmacy counter could complete the amount of work being handed to us. The entire scene was dangerous, and I recognized that.

The biggest problem was the drive-thru. The cars came one after another, making it impossible to spend any time at the counter dispensing drugs. I was literally standing at the window telling each driver that their prescription wasn't ready, so they drove around the building and got back into line, only for me to tell them again that it still wasn't ready because I couldn't return to the dispensing counter. We had six key areas of the pharmacy to staff: drop-off, drive-thru, cash register, phone, dispensing counter, and counseling area. I had to get rid of one of them, so I put an "out of order" sign on the drive-thru just so I could fill prescriptions. It was the one critical point that wasted the most of my time.

I survived the day and teared up while waiting at a red light on the drive home. I had an OBRA-90 meltdown. My head felt like it was about to explode, and my legs were throbbing. Nothing in me agreed with what I had done at work that day, and nothing at all agreed with the way I was being expected to do it. There was only speed, and that was fast. There was no education, no compassion, and no humanity in my work. My mind raced, wondering if I had killed someone, and I was having flashbacks to the dispensing error I'd made while working at another pharmacy under similar conditions. How many computer warnings did I have to blow through while filling prescriptions? How many warnings did my techs push through? Would I soon be facing the paperwork for another dispensing error that I would remember nothing about? For God's sake, the CVS computer screen turned from green to orange to red when you were out of time, and we all knew that the computers reported our numbers to HQ each night. It was the company's way of warning you that you were taking too long to fill a prescription.

As my luck would have it, a customer called CVS headquarters to complain about the "out of order" sign I placed on the drive-thru window. The next day, I received a call from my supervisor, who gave me a tongue-lashing. She explained that she'd had a difficult time saving the job of the last pharmacist who had closed the drive-thru. I thought to myself that she wouldn't need to fight to save mine. I had worked for CVS for barely two months, and I had not yet put my license up on the wall. I was never going to display my state board of pharmacy license having experienced the unprofessional nature of their operations, and never could I "suck it up" and stay there until retirement. My mind was once and for all settled on opening my own business. I gave my notice to quit. My supervisor told me that I need not return, and I was out of there. Good riddance!

Cold feet turned hot, and with this CVS experience leading me to feel that employment in any retail chain would be intolerable, I was now fully committed to opening my own pharmacy. Come hell or high water—and I'd just been through both—this abomination of unprofessionalism was going to drive me forward. It was the easiest resignation of my life and my shortest-lived job, even when compared to my first pharmacy. I chalked up job number ten to being an eye-opening experience and tried my best to forget it. I walked away shaking my head, which was filled with thoughts of what I had tried to accomplish with NAEP, and wondering how things had gotten so bad in the years since I last worked behind the counter of a chain pharmacy. All I could think was, "Who does this? Who in their educated mind does this?" This was yet another part of my employment history that I would leave off my resume if I ever needed to write one again. If I did add it, it would only be in the hope of being asked why my employment at CVS had been so brief.

I lasted long enough at CVS to understand how pharmacist despair can turn into apathy. I felt the pharmacy staff's despair, noticed the skirting of rules, and wondered if I had hurt anyone. I knew that I hadn't helped patients in any significant way beyond perpetuating their false sense of financial benefit or satisfying its insatiable desire to consume.

I am all for companies leveraging economies of scale, purchasing power, and consolidation of labor through information technology. Free-market forces benefit the public, and I understand that. But it's clearly not working out for everyone. Nearly 75 percent of the American public lives paycheck to paycheck, a majority do not have $400 saved for an emergency, and drug misuse and abuse has never before caused so much pain and suffering. From my perspective, CVS's notion of free-market principles meant that everything was free except our time to ensure patient safety, and this notion forced me yet again into the unemployment line. Give me a soup line any day instead of a drive-thru line and a computer screen that changes color according to how long it takes a pharmacist to dispense a prescription for a dangerous drug.

Giant Eagle was looking for a pharmacist at the time, and I was just the right person to fill it because of the hours I was willing to work. Although Giant Eagle was a large retail chain, my friends who worked there had told me that the company provide adequate staffing and did not have an "in your face" computer system that conflicted with a pharmacist's professional discretion. By now, I was refusing to share my resume for fear that potential employers would see my youthful appearance and smile and be stunned by the prospect of being Job Number Eleven. I was straightforward during my interview and told them of my intention to open my own sterile compounding pharmacy. They didn't view this type of pharmacy practice as a threat, and they liked that I was willing to work every evening until close and cover all weekends. I was a manager's dream, giving them evenings and weekends with their families. I began work at the Giant Eagle in Newton Falls immediately and would eventually float to most of the other stores in the area.

I wonder if I set a record, working eleven jobs as a pharmacist in less than twenty years. If anyone else has come close to that, I imagine they probably lost their license at some point along the way. Be that as it may, I was experienced. Except for nuclear pharmacy, I had now worked in just about every practice setting that pharmacy had to offer. I'd worked retail chain (both large and small) and independent pharmacy. I'd worked in hospital pharmacy, home infusion, and long-term care pharmacy. And now, I knew sterile compounding pharmacy. I could dose a TPN, adjust an IV drip, and suck the last drop of drug from a vial. I understood insurance, law, customer service, and the ins and outs of administrative meetings. I was ready to start my own business in the pharmacy world with the knowledge I had taken away from so many pharmacy jobs. Moreover, I could swing a hammer and wire and plumb a house, and I had gathered an assortment of tools to match those of any skilled carpenter. I was finally prepared to roll into the next phase of my life.

Everything about my attitude while working at Giant Eagle was different because I knew I was leaving, and with that, I was able to maintain a bit of enthusiasm during the long days. They offered enough training and seemed to provide plenty of staff to assist me behind the pharmacy counter. Yes, the stores were busy, and I piled up my fair share of baskets, each containing one or more prescription orders, even pausing for a moment to take a picture of the chairs we had to pull up next to the prescription counter because we had run out of room. I had to take the photo quickly, knowing that the eyes of administration were always on us thanks to the cameras that were now popular in the workplace. I didn't care, though. My stay with Giant Eagle was temporary.

I began to look for an empty retail space to open my compounding pharmacy, and that task alone excited me. I was nice to Giant Eagle customers, tolerant of adverse situations, and seemed to not be so tired at the end of the day despite the pace. My enthusiasm made a comeback due to the amount of work I knew I'd have to do to make my business successful. I had the attitude of someone with a purpose when the pharmacists around me were displaying misery and cynicism. This place called retail-chain pharmacy was not my destiny, and just as I had made a clean break from the life of a carney some twenty-five years earlier, I was about to get off a dangerous roller coaster once and for all.

Every chain pharmacy developed ways of circumventing OBRA-90's requirements of gathering information on the front end, conducting a thoughtful DUR, and providing counseling. With each circumvention, they were able to squeeze out a little more profit. A technician would scan a patient's prescription, which would show up in a queue at another pharmacy within the chain miles away. That pharmacy would "do all the work" in "their down time" and send the label back to the originating pharmacy for check-out. Patient refills could be sent to central fill pharmacies to be filled at 2:00 a.m. by pharmacists working on a line; these were then placed in a tote for the next day's delivery to the originating pharmacy. It was becoming increasingly difficult to know who the dispensing pharmacist was, and only the corporate brand remained constant on every label.

I consider myself lucky to have gotten out just before the added burdens of administering vaccines were dumped on the shoulders of chain pharmacists. Pharmacy associations like OPA and APhA supported and even pushed for this development, as they saw the service as an additional revenue stream that would help make up for money lost to insurance companies. APhA began its first nationally recognized immunization in 1996, and although it would take a decade or so to become a widespread practice in retail pharmacies, the added burden eventually arrived. It was a heavy burden for those who already had precious little time to dedicate to anything other than making sure the right pills were in the right bottle.

The year was 2006. According to the CDC it was the year that marked the beginning of a steady increase in overall national opioid dispensing rates. It was also the year when government received its first warning about "disturbing data" showing an uptick in addiction rates. The data was flagged by the directors of the National Institute on Drug Abuse and the National Institute of Health. Apparently, it was our nation's rate of obesity and the growth of meth labs that pushed this warning to the backburner. A study in 2005 that showed one in ten high school students had abused Vicodin, an opioid painkiller containing hydrocodone, was the canary that could have brought attention to OBRA-90 adherence. Instead, retail chain pharmacy was doing as retail chain pharmacy does, and the pharmacists working for them were caught in a never-ending cycle of unprofessionalism. Our first opportunity to nip the opioid crisis in the butt came and went in 2006 without OBRA-90 being considered as a fix.

◆ ◆ ◆

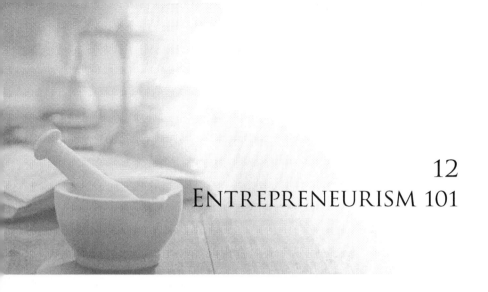

12
ENTREPRENEURISM 101

Uncle Ray had bequeathed me thirty acres of property in North Kingsville, Ohio, near Lake Erie, and I used it as collateral to obtain seed money to open my compounding pharmacy. I began searching for a place to set up shop, and by January of 2007, I'd found one in Poland, Ohio. It was set back from the road a bit but on busy Route 224, which connects Poland with Boardman and Canfield. It was one section of a four-section plaza, and I signed the lease on my wife's birthday. I had $40,000 in the bank and immediately began chipping away at it. The nine-hundred-square-foot space needed to contain an anteroom, a cleanroom, an office, and a customer seating area.

As an entrepreneur, one of the most exciting parts of the journey is when you sit down with a pen and pad of paper and begin to brainstorm names for your new business. I did a quick internet search thanks to this new engine called Google and found that the name RC Compounding Services had not yet been taken. After filing the necessary application with the Secretary of State, I was now the owner of a compounding pharmacy. There was much to do, and I was excited to have taken these first big steps. They're the part of the journey that determines who will run their own business and who will continue working for others.

The expertise I'd gained from my previous eleven jobs, combined with my carpentry skills, made my $40,000 seem like $400,000. I plastered, painted, laid flooring, and wired all the equipment necessary to provide a clean space to mix compounded drugs. For several months, I ended my day at RC Compounding (RCC) at 4:00 p.m., changed my cloths, put on a tie, and had just enough time to drive to the Giant Eagle in Newton Falls, about forty-five minutes away, where I worked until closing. Then, I got up the next day and did the whole thing over again. I got small breaks on the weekends when days at Giant Eagle were short, and I could spend time with my family at home. I was a carpenter by day and a pharmacist at night, spending money just as fast as I was making it.

Once the dirty work of physically building RCC was done, I began to make things look pretty in the office and waiting area. I needed a logo, business cards, brochures, and, crucially, a license from the Ohio Board of Pharmacy. I received my Employer Identification Number, Worker's Comp number, National Provider Number, and wholesaler account, and I purchased a basic prescription filling program from the cheapest vendor I could find. My $40,000 had now dwindled to $10,000, and I still needed to buy drugs and supplies.

A compounding-supply company called Medisca not only allowed me to purchase the drugs and supplies I needed, but it also gave me technical support on best practices to make drug dosages accurate. I was already good at working with intrathecal syringes, and their guidance helped me expand into other areas of drug compounding. This partnership continues today, despite the number of other companies that would later enter the industry and bid for my business.

Medisca consumed the last of my money, and in May of 2007, I was able to tell my anxious wife that I was ready to open for business. She was handling almost everything at home in my absence, and although she was happy to hear that the business was coming along, I still had to work evenings and weekends at Giant Eagle. It would be weeks before my first official sale; a consistent revenue stream high enough to be considered an income was a year away. My posted hours of operation at RCC still reads "8:00 AM–4:00 PM," even though we're now open until 4:30. I just don't have the heart to change it.

For the longest time, I hoped the phone would ring, if it was just a wrong number. I prayed someone would walk in, even if only to ask for directions. Even though the average citizen had no need for a sterile intrathecal syringe of drugs, I was looking for company. All I had was my dad next to me, and as precious as he was in helping get my business off the ground, I'd heard all his stories and advice several times over. I finally made my first deposit in my business bank account in June of 2007. It was for $150, and I have that receipt framed in my office.

What I provided was not a drug that just anyone could walk in and purchase. I was compounding sterile intrathecal syringes for use in pain pumps, and my clientele were physicians. Although I no longer compound drugs for use in the spine and no longer have controlled substances like morphine on my shelf, the type of pharmacy product that I offered when I first opened involves weighing out the pure powdered drug, dissolving that drug in water, and filtering it to remove any contaminants. Sometimes, these drugs can be sterilized in an oven, but one way or another, they need to be clean. The risk of infection is always present because the drug is considered "dirty" to begin with, and because of this risk, very few pharmacies in the country provide this type of product.

I needed to hit the road and visit physicians' offices if I wanted to drum up business. I would set my store alarm, lock the doors, and drive to physicians' offices, where my top goal was getting the nurse behind the sliding glass window to talk to me. I purchased a couple cases of shiny folders with my name and logo—an $800 bill I couldn't afford—and jumped into my disgusting-looking black four-door Mercury Tracer. Given the delicacy and expertise of my trade, I was careful to park well away from the clinics I visited so as not to be vehicularly associated with what I was trying to sell.

Few in our state had the knowledge or courage to mix a drug, most often an opioid, from a non-sterile, or "dirty," powder and prepare it in such a way as to be safe for administration into the spine. This area, like the brain, has zero tolerance for bacteria. Contamination from either air or touch would result in meningitis and possible death. The laws, regulations, agency oversight, and even literature governing this practice were all lacking back then, but I policed myself, knowing the consequences. I spent weeks writing my own standard operating procedures and sought accreditation by the recently formed Pharmacy Compounding Accreditation Board (PCAB). I would later become an inspector for PCAB until my business grew large enough to steal what little free time I had. RC Compounding Services, LLC, was the first compounding pharmacy in Ohio to receive PCAB accreditation.

I always had this sense that the business would be okay. I tried to reassure my wife and thanked her for shouldering much of the burden of raising our three active children during that first intense year. During times of obsession—like opening a new business—our passion-filled tunnel vision can prevent us from appreciating the efforts of others around us. The oversight that cuts the deepest is when those who love you most and those you love most become blurry images in this tunnel vision. Throw into the mix the anxiety of a past business failure, job changes every year or two, and a checkbook balance reading zero, and you can imagine the steep climb a new business owner needs to make and why so few attempt it. Lori was now a full-time math instructor at Youngstown State University, and she sorted out the numbers and explained to me what was on each side of the equal sign. If I ever gave her the impression that she seemed blurry to me, she would quickly clarify that image.

Being the college math instructor that my wife is, and due to our previous experience with debt and interest payments, she forbid the purchase of any drugs, supplies, or equipment unless we were able to pay for it. This was one of the most important business decisions she made for us, and since she was aware of my spending habits, she held firm as the CFO of RC Compounding and set us on a track to financial stability. She knew that if the business failed, we would walk away with hurt feelings and wasted energy, but no debt. We had just experienced the 2008 financial meltdown, when banks teetered on the edge of collapse, and we were both leery of the lending institutions that didn't seem to be making loans anyway.

As the months passed, I changed my schedule at Giant Eagle and stopped working nights. I continued working weekends to supplement my income, but after a few months of that, I asked that they call me in only when they really needed someone to fill in. The pharmacist shortage was coming to an end in 2008, so I had a feeling they wouldn't be needing me. I was now able to give 100 percent to RC Compounding, and for the second time in my life, I was my own boss. But this time, it looked as though I just might stay that way.

One day, I received a call from a nurse at a local eye clinic, asking if I was able to prepare a particular kind of sterile syringe that they used a lot. They used it to inject a drug directly into the eye, and no mixing needed to be done on my part. I simply had to draw up the drug directly from a vial, label it, bag it, and deliver it to their office. They would attach their own needle prior to giving their patients the injection. "Why not just draw it up yourself?" I thought. It turned out that the vial cost a couple thousand dollars, and after taking one very small dose needed to administer to a patient, the rest of the drug that remained in the vial would have to be tossed out. The drug was called Avastin, and after a bit of research, I headed to their office to see what this type of administration was all about.

A tumor produces a protein called VEGF, and this protein stimulates the formation of capillaries from which it will draw its blood supply and feed. If a person has several tumors, the dominant tumor will produce higher quantities of this protein and thus become the dominant tumor within the host. Avastin is an anti-VEGF medication used to treat cancer by blocking the formation of these blood vessels that feed various tumors.

Macular degeneration is an overgrowth of capillaries in the back of the eye where the retina is located, and it is one of the leading causes of blindness in the U.S. This overgrowth of blood vessels eventually crowds out the retina and prevents light from reaching it. Physicians began injecting just a couple of drops of Avastin directly into the vitreous of the eye and saw astonishing results. Blindness due to macular degeneration finally had an effective treatment! There was just one problem: Avastin was not commercially available in small doses for use in the eye. It was available in 4 milliliter ($800) and 16 milliliter ($3200) vials that could only be punctured once by a needle. The drug is normally used to treat colon cancer, so to obtain many small, affordable doses, the eye clinic needed to turn to a sterile compounding pharmacy.

I studied how the individual syringes were labeled, packaged, and stored. It all seemed simple enough, and after a period of study and preparation, I was repackaging Avastin for physician administration. My first orders were going out, and money was finally coming in. I had a new product, and things were looking up for me. My cold calls to Youngstown, Akron, and Cleveland eye clinics were bringing in accounts, and I was learning more about an industry that still seemed to be in its nascent stage. We had USP and PCAB to guide us, but actual laws with rules and regulations were only just being discussed. This laxity in the laws allowed some pharmacies that were compounding sterile drugs to continue doing so in back warehouses or closet-like rooms where cases of paper towels were being stored. Tragedy had thus far escaped our industry, but it wouldn't for much longer.

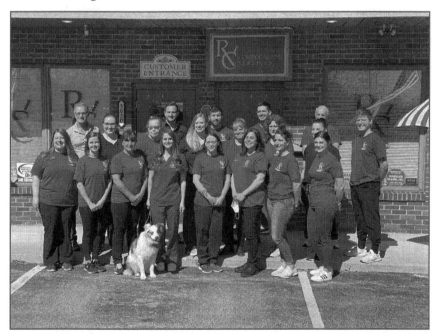

Staff at RC Compounding Services

❖ ❖ ❖

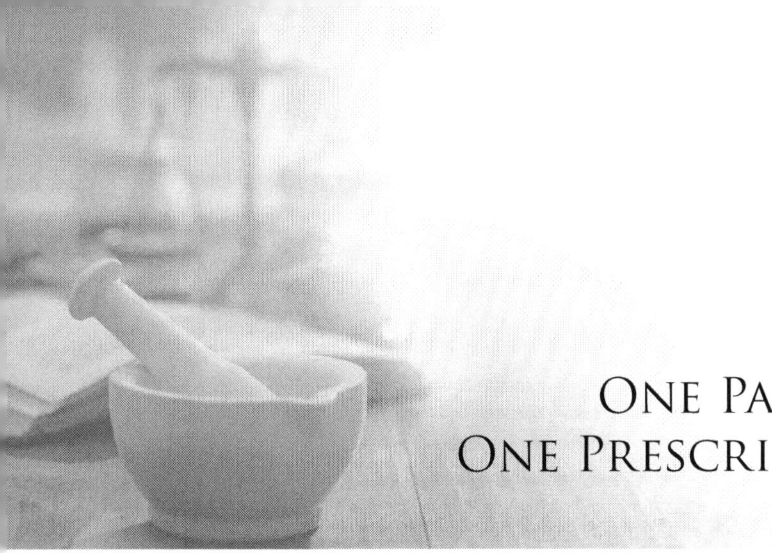

13
One Patient, One Prescription

My interactions with the Ohio Board of Pharmacy had been similar to those of most pharmacists. Do no wrongs, and you will receive no visits. Receiving only a Terminal of Dangerous Drug Distributors license prior to opening a pharmacy would guarantee a visit by a Board of Pharmacy inspector. If the Board inspector liked what they saw, the new pharmacy owner was handed their license to operate and could commence pharmacy-related activities—and not a moment before then. This is different from dealing with the FDA, which, in certain instances, allows operations to begin after an application is received.

Ohio is a tough state to practice pharmacy in, and other pharmacists around the country recognize this fact.

The inspector in my area was Joann Predina, and even though I was never allowed to say that I liked her, I did. Of course, I would be lying if I said I liked her the first time we met. She came into the pharmacies I had worked in previously, sometimes unannounced, and wasted no time in grilling me on the hows and whys of whatever I was doing. She accepted no beverages, no snacks, and rarely a compliment without giving a scowl. She was there to ply her trade, not fraternize or sugarcoat what the people expected of us. She gave me my first true inspection as a pharmacist, and I was somewhat defensive of the constructive criticism she gave our department.

I would later be inspected five or six times by the FDA at two locations—perhaps a record for an individual pharmacist—and I would come to appreciate the way Joann prepared me. She's also the one who put my name in the hat to become a PCAB inspector. There are few people today whom I have come to respect more than Joann Predina for the professional direction she has given me. She could look past my eyes and into my professional brain to scold me if she sensed I was creeping too far into the moral hazards of pharmacy practice. I never wanted to stray due to the respect I had for her and the punishment I knew I would deserve if I crossed the line.

My sense of what was expected of me as a pharmacist was grounded in my professional association days and the hours I spent typing up bylaws for various groups. In my mind, learned people got together in a room and hashed out the best way to ensure that things would run smoothly without causing harm to patients. It didn't matter to me if they were referring to the duties of the pharmacist in charge or the way a pharmacy technician was supposed to clean a refrigerator. The more direction I was given, the less ambiguity there was to my activities or the activities of those working for me. These rules kept me safe and out of court. Plus, I had a business reason to comply with the rules.

Many pharmacists in compounding fought tooth and nail against rules and regulations, constantly complained that the rules were unreasonable, and argued that they had been doing this stuff for years without incident. "No one's getting hurt" and "This is just how we've always done it" seemed to be the attitude of many pharmacists in our industry. Some were so headstrong that they even refused to allow FDA inspectors into their pharmacy. They clung to some vague interpretation of the law that they didn't have to allow federal agents on their premises because their pharmacy was regulated by their state Board of Pharmacy. When the federal agents returned with a warrant signed by a judge, it meant these pharmacists had only made things worse for themselves. Sticking to their guns meant that they might eventually cease to exist as a legitimate operation.

For me, this meant more business. I was happy to have one hundred new rules to follow because my competition would accept only ten before handing their business over to me. I'd spent years studying Ohio pharmacy law so I could uncover new services that the people wanted from me and protect those that I was already serving. The law represented the people's point of view, and their interests mattered more than the pharmacy's.

I didn't seem to have to worry about a Board of Pharmacy rule that limits how much a pharmacy is able to sell to customers without a physician's prescription. A pharmacy in Ohio that is licensed and overseen by the Ohio Board of Pharmacy is free to fill as many prescriptions as they want so long as a physician has written orders for each one of them. This means that a patient's name is attached to the bottle containing the drug and that the bottle is handed directly to the patient. If you want to sell a compounded drug like Avastin without a patient name on a label, sales of these wholesale-like transactions cannot exceed 5 percent of your annual sales.

At first, my fledgling pharmacy didn't have many sales, so I skipped this section, knowing that I was way below the limits set in the rules. But as RC Compounding's sales increased, so did my attention to this rule. More and more of what I was compounding and selling—specifically, Avastin—was for "office use only." This was a wholesale transaction, and I was not a licensed wholesaler.

RC Compounding was a specialty retail pharmacy first, and I had to follow the same Board rules as places like CVS and Walgreens. We all held the same Terminal Distributor of Dangerous Drug license. My problem was that I was compounding all the drugs I dispensed, and my pharmacy acted more like a manufacturer than a CVS or Walgreens that held the same license. Offices and clinics would call to order fifty doses of a drug, but they couldn't provide fifty individual prescriptions for individual patients. The rules as written were preventing this public need from being met. And this need within our communities was growing exponentially.

The purpose behind this rule was to maintain what our profession calls the "triad." The triad refers to the physician, pharmacist, and patient relationship, which is held together by what is known as "dispensing pursuant to a patient prescription." Having a single name on a vial of drugs means that if a mistake occurs, only one patient will be injured. Sending out fifty doses of a compounded drug to a clinic means that fifty patients could be injured if there's an error. This is why we have separate licenses for pharmacies, wholesalers, and manufacturers, but times were changing, and public need was changing. Society was making "new discoveries," as Jefferson put it, and compounding pharmacy fell somewhere between understood and under-defined.

Losing the triad relationship between pharmacist, physician, and patient might accelerate the rate of drug misuse and abuse. Unfortunately, chain and mail-order pharmacies looking to increase sales pushed aside the rules that all but demanded that this relationship be maintained, one prescription and one patient name at a time. The triad was overwhelmed by numbers, speed, and metrics, and no relationship can exist between the different parties of the triad unless they spend time fostering it. When my Board of Pharmacy inspector explained this safety concept to me, I wondered why it was not being enforced in the chain setting.

Despite my belief in the inherent good to be found in the triad, there was a growing need for wholesale drugs without patient names attached. Drug shortages were peaking, and surgical centers were popping up on every corner. I emailed the Board with my concerns about the 5 percent rule, made several phone calls, invited then-State Senator Shiavoni to my business to discuss the issue, and emailed my state association, the Ohio Pharmacists Association. This rule needed to be re-examined and perhaps rewritten.

I was receiving patient-specific orders for drugs that would never end up in the hands of patients and would instead be directly administered by physicians in their offices and clinics. We struggled with the labor-intensive need to keep names straight, set delivery times, and toss drugs when a patient's dose was not needed because an appointment was cancelled. Clinics were upset that they had to write individual prescriptions. And all this extra, unnecessary work was taking our focus away from critical duties, like ensuring that our cleanroom was indeed clean. Our customers frequently told us that "so-and-so pharmacy doesn't require us to provide them with prescriptions," and this meant that I was losing business to com-pounding pharmacies located in other states.

I made a total of three trips to Columbus to meet with our Board of Pharmacy executive director and staff regarding this 5 percent rule. When the Ohio Board of Pharmacy Rules Review Committee finally met, I was present and handed them my written request for review. I petitioned the committee to look at changes occurring in healthcare, with patients undergoing surgical procedures outside of hospitals. These centers had drug needs that were being met by pharmacies in other states, which our BOP was unable to inspect.

The Rules Review Committee responded by tabling my petition because they felt they "lacked expertise in the area," and the BOP executive director told me that I would be placed on the next committee to offer an alternative to the 5 percent rule. There was nothing more they could do, and if I wanted to continue selling drugs to clinics without a patient name, I would have to register with the Food and Drug Administration as a "Repacker of Sterile Drugs."

Okay, I could do that. I researched what I had to do to apply, hired a consultant to help link my computer with the FDA's, and transmitted my application.

With some FDA licenses, an applicant can begin operations as soon as the FDA receives their application. The FDA must assume that the applicant has not only hired consultants, but also lawyers, engineers, and past regulatory agents and that they're confident in their level of FDA compliance to begin business in lieu of an actual FDA inspection. I submitted my application and immediately notified the Ohio Board of Pharmacy that I had registered as a repacker with the FDA and that I was preparing orders without patient prescriptions in that capacity. This move, I thought, would buy me some time, but only if that time allowed for a change to Ohio's 5 percent rule.

Unfortunately, time was not going to wait for me. A moral hazard was just around the corner, and it was being perpetrated by another compounding pharmacy in another state that was making big profits and risking patient safety while they did so. My appointment to our board of pharmacy Rules Review Committee never happened, and all conversations about who was a wholesaler and who was a pharmacy ground to a halt because of the reckless behavior of an out-of-state compounding pharmacy, too far away from our state to inspect, that was putting Donald Duck-like names on the drugs they were shipping across state lines.

I mention this thing called a "moral hazard" several times because events that were about to unfold in our world of compounding pharmacy were directly tied to this concept. There is a difference between committing an unlawful act and committing a moral hazard. One is obvious and the other is not. One is illegal and the other, immoral. And if an act is deemed illegal, it must have a law in place to declare it such. Consequently, a moral hazard has no legal precedent and therefore is looked at only as an immoral act. Either, when committed, can bring about similar levels of pain and suffering to those against whom the act was committed.

According to Britannica, a moral hazard is the risk one party incurs when dependent on the moral behavior of others. The risk increases when there is no effective way to control that behavior or when there is an incentive to misbehave. The incentive for one party to misbehave is greatly increased when the other party to the transaction is ignorant of the terms and rules guiding the behavior.

The world of compounding had few definitive laws guiding its practice, and immoral individuals would take advantage of the fact that policing agencies like our boards of pharmacy and the FDA has "no effective way to control" their behavior. They were willing to take a risk because there was little in law that said they could act a particular way, and in doing so, people would die. Agencies would swoop in and look for a way to lawfully control behavior, new laws would be written, and laws that once needed only one hundred words to guide the behavior of moral individuals would become one thousand words to rein in the immoral.

This concept must be considered in the world of retail chain pharmacy, knowing that OBRA-90 laws are already in place, so that we can understand how and why our nation's opioid epidemic began. Compounding pharmacy in 2012 was in its infancy, and retail pharmacy was not. The damage done is the same when the offense is perpetrated by individuals who look to skirt the law, claim no law exists, or rely on a public that is ignorant of the law feel safe enough to take the risk of being caught. Corporate pharmacy chains looked for whatever grey areas of the law they could find, they read between lines, and came up with their own definitions of "reasonable attempt" so they could remove the time their pharmacists could spend on patient care and give it to the gimmicks that would allow them to increase customer volume and profitability.

◆ ◆ ◆

14
AN AGENCY CAN ACT
WHEN TRAGEDY STRIKES

DURING THE SEPTEMBER 2012 presidential debate between Barack Obama and Mitt Romney on national TV, an emergency message began to scroll along the bottom of the screen. Patients in several states had been hospitalized with meningitis and more were on their way to the hospital. Some had already died from it.

Meningitis is an excruciatingly painful way to lose your life, and when it's caused by a fungus, it can be very difficult to treat. Fungi are slow to grow, slow to result in symptoms after injection because of this growth rate, and difficult to kill because it eats the anti-fungal meds slowly. Drugs that are typically used to kill fungal infections need to be administered in high doses for long periods of time, and those who survive endure intense pain in the brain and spinal column.

For the next several weeks, the number of patients who were either sick or dead increased steadily, and the CDC and FDA worked feverishly to find the source. It was soon traced back to three lots of supposedly sterile vials of methylprednisolone for injection that were compounded by a pharmacy in Massachusetts.

Methylprednisolone is a steroid delivered via epidural injection to reduce inflammation in patients with back pain, and in 2012, the manufacturers of the drug, Pfizer and Teva, were finding it difficult to keep up with demand—and they were the only two companies manufacturing it. Clinics and physicians' offices that wanted to treat their patients with this steroid had no choice but to order it from compounding pharmacies. Although the law states that such facilities are not allowed to compound drugs that are already commercially available from an FDA-approved manufacturer, drug shortages allowed for exceptions.

I tried to compound this drug at RC Compounding, but it was soon clear that the FDA would deem it beyond the scope of our facility. We didn't have the right equipment, so I stopped compounding it. Methylprednisolone doesn't dissolve into a solution but is rather a suspension of floating particles that settle to the bottom of the vial during heat sterilization, and even the most experienced compounders need advanced mixing equipment. The final vial must be sterilized in an oven or autoclave to kill any bacteria, mold, or fungus that may have entered it during compounding.

The compounding pharmacy responsible for the contaminated drugs was the New England Compounding Center (NECC) in Massachusetts. It had falsified cleaning logs, ignored filth growing in and near its cleanrooms, and failed to test each lot for sterility before releasing it to the public.

In the end, over seventy-five patients lost their lives, and another seven hundred were sickened by these contaminated vials, which had been shipped to seventy-six facilities in twenty-three states. The owner of the company would eventually be sent to prison for eight years.

What happens within a state stays in the state, but as soon as you cross state lines and enter the realm of interstate commerce, you're in federal territory overseen by the FDA. Congress responded to this tragedy by passing a new law, the Drug Quality and Security Act (DQSA), in November of 2013. From that moment on, compounding pharmacies were a leaf in the governmental stream. Even though I played no part in the error myself, RCC and the rest of the compounding pharmacy world would have to pay the penance, and we were holding our collective breaths, hoping we would be allowed to operate at all, given what had just happened.

My timing was poor because I was a compounding pharmacy that had just applied to become a repacker of sterile drugs. In effect, what I had submitted just before the NECC tragedy was an invitation to the FDA to inspect my sterile compounding pharmacy when they were looking for easy access to such facilities, and since, in my mind, they were higher on the agency food chain than our Board of Pharmacy, I was not about to turn them away when they flashed their badges.

A part of me hoped that my application had failed to go through, was disregarded, or had gotten lost somewhere in the data oblivion that I had paid so much in consulting fees to enter. Instead, the Food and Drug Administration walked in on February 2, 2013, months before the law was passed, and flashed their badges. They were accompanied by Joann Predina of the Ohio Board of Pharmacy. I suspect that mine was the first compounding pharmacy in Ohio to be inspected by the FDA after the NECC tragedy.

The FDA agents came dressed in uniforms with briefcases and computers in hand, and despite their intimidating appearance, they were very professional. I felt very distant from them in the sense that they were not from around here, not from Ohio, and all we shared was our president of the United States. Oddly, it was comforting having an inspector from our Board of Pharmacy present.

The FDA agents spent five days collecting information and giving me my first taste of what it was like to be inspected by a federal agency. In the end, I was given a form by the FDA that rescinded my application to operate as a sterile drug repacker, and I went back to filling patient-specific prescriptions under Ohio law. Since the NECC contamination had happened just months earlier, there were no lawful provision on the books to allow compounding pharmacies to dispense in any way other than one patient-one prescription.

It was a very emotional experience for me, and I choked up a bit during our "exit meeting." I had fought tooth and nail, asking our Board of Pharmacy to allow those compounding pharmacies that they could inspect to safely produce and sell the kinds of products that caused this situation in the first place. The two years I had spent writing this warning and traveling to deliver it had become one big "I told you so," and unfortunately, I was about to pay the same hefty price as other compounders. Joann was present for this meeting, and she was sympathetic to my situation; she was aware of my prior efforts.

While I felt that my PCAB accreditation made my compounding pharmacy processes better than most, it was clear that we still had deficiencies. According to the FDA, compounding drugs and selling them without a physician prescription made you more of a manufacturer than a pharmacy, and they expected a level of care that followed their Code of Federal Regulations (CFR). This CFR-level of time and investment was not practical in a pharmacy setting and cost millions of dollars that only true manufacturers could afford, so they eventually established a middle-ground for compounding pharmacies. These FDA expectations are called "guidance documents," and although they are non-binding recommendations and contain only the "current thinking of the FDA," we bind them together in a folder and put them on the shelf next to our law books.

The confusion, disruptions, added costs, and loss of customers meant that I had to let one of my pharmacists—my best friend,

Jon, with whom I'd worked at St. Joe's and whom I had hired when things were looking up—go. He was an expensive employee, and I simply couldn't afford him. It was an ugly end to a great relationship. I purchased his half of the cabin that we owned together, and we never really talked again. The world was changing, and we had to change with it, especially now that the Feds were determining who we would become.

I like to think that RC Compounding may have helped to shape our new DQSA law, thanks to what the FDA agents may or may not have seen during our inspection. We certainly had to be one of the first to be inspected after the NEC tragedy unfolded. Our commitment to following the rules and suggesting new ones was on display throughout the week the FDA spent with us, and although we had our share of deficiencies, most came from grey areas of the law that had yet to be made clear. Our industry was about to get the agency attention we deserved, and the guidance that would soon be written would add clarity to our activities. RC Compounding demonstrated that we understood what needed to be done and the reasons why, and this was made possible by a pharmacist's education that pulled from various subjects.

The new federal law gave the FDA oversight of office-use compounded drugs, while individual state pharmacy boards would oversee patient-specific dispensing of compounded prescriptions. Each state needed to sign a "Memorandum of Understanding," just to be sure that the relationship between the FDA and the States was clear.

This law created a new category of pharmacy practice called "Outsourcing Facilities," and anyone who wanted to sell compounded drugs without a prescription from a physician would need to register as one with the FDA. We would be half-pharmacy and half-manufacturer in that we would be able to make and sell fifty or one hundred doses of a drug for a physician to use in their office with a simple phone call or fax request. We still needed a license from the Ohio BOP, but they would have limited oversight.

This law was not as lengthy as some other pieces of legislation Congress has been known to pass, but it was long enough to tell us where we stood. Given the tragic outcome of the error made by the New England Compounding Center, the number of citizens who had died or gotten sick, and the filth the FDA found while inspecting NECC's facility, you can imagine how happy we were that the law would allow us to continue doing business—and that it mandated that a pharmacist should oversee it.

It was thanks to the efforts of APhA, NCPA, ICPA, and other pharmacy organizations that we were spared—democracy at work! Best of all, the FDA published their guidance outlining what we had to do as a pharmacy and what we did not have to do as a manufacturer, and these guidelines were appropriate and reasonable. They could have made testing requirements and operational procedures so expensive as to prohibit us from caring for customers at all. We had our hands full, but we still had our work, which could have easily been taken from us and given to another profession. We had dodged a bullet!

Wanting to comply with the new law as quickly as possible, I immediately filed an application with the FDA to register as an Outsourcing Facility and paid the $12,000 fee. I created a new company called RC Outsourcing (RCO) and proceeded to do business under the same roof as RC Compounding. I would simply keep all records separate between the two. The new rule that the two types of businesses needed to be in separate locations wasn't clear, and I jumped the gun instead of waiting for additional guidance.

Low and behold, shortly thereafter, the FDA published "For Entities Considering Whether To Register As Outsourcing Facilities

Under Section 503B of the Federal Food, Drug, and Cosmetic Act."
It was now clear that I would have to move the wholesale part of my
business, build a new cleanroom, reapply at a new location, and pay
another $12,000 fee. My wife was ready to kill me, and I knew better
than to plead for an exception, so I began to look for a second location
to house a second business. Now that I had experienced both FDA
and BOP inspections of sterile compounding, I was determined to
stay in the game. I just needed to know the rules I had to follow, and
although many rules were still a work in progress by both agencies,
I had enough to go on.

Our hometown's downtown area looks much like the other
downtowns in the surrounding communities. The steel mills that
once operated just upriver from Lowellville and continued into
surrounding communities had rusted away or been dismantled
entirely and sold for scrap. The downtown areas that were once
enriched by the economic activity of steel making now consist of
mostly abandoned and boarded-up buildings. One such empty building in our hometown was our local bank, which sat prominently
in the middle of town next to a big green bridge that crossed the
Mahoning River.

The Lowellville Savings and Loan building, complete with safes,
vaults, and thick walls, was empty and for sale. I thought it would
suit our needs for an FDA-registered facility. It was a safe and secure
fortress with teller windows and a basement that flooded each time it
rained. I would have my hands full turning this into an outsourcing
facility, and knowing that Lori wouldn't allow us to incur any debt in
this endeavor, I'd have to do the renovations myself with our limited
funds. I purchased the old bank and began to renovate it in May of
2015. I missed out on much of our popular Lowellville Festival that
summer, spending most of that period in the basement fixing drainage

problems. That done, I moved upstairs to gut the teller windows, restore the beautiful vaults, and build a top-notch cleanroom.

By the end of the summer, I had everything certified and ready for the FDA and Ohio Board of Pharmacy inspections. My sign was erected on the façade, and I added hunter-green awnings above each window. The building looked nice both inside and out. We were ready with our operating procedures, equipment, and trained staff to begin business and put this chapter behind us.

Our Ohio Board of Pharmacy inspection seemed to go well, although no one is ever given the liberty to claim so. It's a process filled with anxiety and anticipation. From the state's perspective, much was still unclear, from the type of license we would hold to how they would coordinate oversight of our activities with the FDA. We knew one thing, though: we wouldn't be able to begin doing business without a state inspector's approval.

Joann Predina handed me my license as she left, and with that, I was now the proud owner of an FDA-licensed outsourcing facility. This was the last time we would interact professionally, as she retired shortly thereafter. This new pharmacy practice setting probably gave me the record for most varied pharmacy experience—if I didn't already hold it. But now, my wife appreciated what my past employment had given me.

We were one of only about sixty outsourcing facilities at the time, which was quite an accomplishment for me and my staff. Even more impressive, we were a "mom and pop" operation in the middle of Lowellville, Ohio, yet competing with big players from around the country.

The old bank building is located just across the street from my failed Carlson's Riverside Pharmacy, so it made my grand opening all the sweeter. Because an outsourcing facility has a different business model than a walk-in pharmacy, I didn't have to rely on the citizens of Lowellville to patronize it. I already had my customers. There weren't many yet, but I believed that I would be able to increase my business as other sterile compounders dropped out of the field.

When others balk at our ideas or ambitions, I ask them, "Why not us?" We have every ability and every right to do the same things that others do. We can put Lowellville, Ohio, on the map, just as others have done for their hometowns. Plus, we had already done things that others had not. We spoke out about the issues facing our industry two years before anyone else.

RCO was now licensed by the State of Ohio and ready for the FDA to inspect us. I gave our team a pep talk to prepare them mentally for the Feds' visit.

RC Outsourcing LLC's first FDA inspection was now a familiar process. They showed their badges and stayed with us for a week or so, collecting detailed information and analyzing every aspect of everything we did. There was no hiding, no misleading, and no circumventing what they wanted to see. My outsourcing facility was small compared to others that made a litany of difficult-to-compound drugs. In contrast, we were basically just repacking a sterile drug that was already commercially available and already sterile. Even so, when compounding sterile drugs for human consumption, things can go wrong—terribly wrong—and so, we endured their fastidious activities, knowing the goal was safety.

I suppose it's possible for a facility to be inspected and not receive what the FDA calls "observations," but it's unlikely, and we always felt good if we managed to keep ours to single digits. After we received these "observations," which are simply those things that the FDA wants changed, we had fifteen business days to respond with our proposed fix. Once we mailed our reply to the agency, we simply had to wait for a response. Sometimes, weeks, months, or even a year could pass before we received a follow-up from them.

That follow-up sometimes took the form of a warning letter if the FDA believed a facility didn't really understand what was being asked of it. This correspondence seemed more threatening in nature. It was the FDA's way of offering further incentive to act and was one step away from a court injunction if they felt it was necessary. We all had sweaty palms when we responded to a warning letter, because we knew this was public information. Such a letter from the FDA reflected poorly on us, even if we thought there was a misunderstanding about what they saw or how we explained our fix.

Some drugs were too complicated to mix and involved too many risky activities for us to comfortably take on. These would have required us to institute procedures that were more akin to procedures carried out by actual drug manufacturers. We were not that and were happy to repackage already commercially available drugs that had received FDA assurances further upstream. We compounded drugs that were already sterile, using supplies that were already sterilized for us. RC Outsourcing's business model was not without risk, but we stayed away from compounding drugs that seemed riskier than others.

Between 2012 and 2015, we saw that when agencies want to address concerns about patient safety, they can bring about change quickly. New laws were passed, and inspectors came in with computers and checklists to ensure that anyone playing in that space was abiding by the rules. There was a new professional assertiveness. Checklists were followed, and reports were written and posted for public display. If someone wanted to argue with the new guidelines, they could expect an injunction from a judge, a recall of their product, or a public lashing on a government site that would dissuade potential customers from using their business.

Uncle Sam can respond with fury, and if there were times when it seemed like the Feds took their sweet time to respond, it only accentuated the anxieties that moved our company to action. The transformation our industry underwent could and should occur in retail-chain pharmacy to protect patient safety as well, if only these agencies could discern the harm they were causing.

Prior to 2012, the laws governing compounding were minimal and vague, and agencies had to train inspectors to enforce them once they were written. Contrast this with retail pharmacy dispensing laws that were already on the books and trained agency staff that was knowledgeable of them. I can only scratch my head as to why workplace conditions in retail-chain pharmacies are not being addressed as a safety concern. Somehow, the resultant suffering either escapes our agencies' attention or they are guided by bias from within the profession itself. Maybe they aren't being guided at all, and the suffering is simply the result of continued silence among those stakeholders who hope the new normal can last until their period of employment ends. Who cares about public sustainability if there's a gold parachute or tenure in place?

In the same year that the NECC tragedy happened, doses of opioids dispensed finally leveled off, and heroin overdoses at the hands of "street pharmacists" began to rise. We were able to see cause and effect in sterile compounding, so if the FDA is able to recognize death at the hands of an immoral pharmacist who spent more time counting money than cleaning his IV hoods, why can't they recognize opioid deaths at the hands of immoral chain pharmacies that demand pharmacists spend more time signing customers up for an auto-refill APPs than counseling patients on the dangers of the drugs they are about to consume? Is it because the death is not as easily attributable to a cause, or is only compounding pharmacy in agency purview and not retail pharmacy?

Understanding how the FDA and boards of pharmacy brought patient safety to compounding pharmacy, one can only wonder why such an organized system of response could not be mobilized against retail chain pharmacy. Given the staggering numbers of citizens dying from medication misuse, from where will the impetus to act come, if not from these deaths alone? The moral hazard perpetrated by an individual who refused to make his cleanroom sterile resulted in direct death and was deemed unlawful. He did prison time as a result. Failing to make a reasonable attempt to capture patient information when a prescription is handed to a pharmacist, or asking a customer "do you have any questions for the pharmacist" in order to avoid taking the time to properly counsel, must not be so obvious a patient safety violation for the FDA to act, if in fact they are the agency that should act.

So, okay, I will institute a form for my sterile technicians to complete every day that documents that our floors were witnessed being wet for the five-minute contact time it takes a disinfecting solution to be effective; and do not require a chain pharmacist to document the number of days that saw patient counseling times total less than ten minutes when those days' prescriptions exceeded three hundred. Go figure?

We have a misallocation of agency resources because there is no legislative directive, and there is no legislative directive because there is no obviousness to the cause and effects of not following OBRA-90. If the law said that a pharmacist must obtain twelve bits of patient information at the time a prescription was dropped off, and pharmacists obtained only five as they do today, that would be unlawful. But because the law states that a pharmacist must make a reasonable attempt, it's just immoral to obtain anything less. Death is death, drugs are drugs, and only the public can pressure legislators to consider that five out of twelve is not reasonable during an opioid epidemic.

I sat back in amazement of how swiftly and decisively our federal and state agencies changed compounding pharmacy between 2013–2015. And I could not help but to think that all I had endured over that short period of time was all that chain pharmacy needed to endure. Nothing happens in a day when problems are complex. New rules emerge and new guidance published as new revelations about the industry are discovered, but it all begins by recognizing that a problem exists. When people are dying, agencies are given the authority to make changes to some of the freedoms that the immoral had abused. As I saw it, this entire process of professional and lawful accountability needed brought to the doorsteps of corporate chain pharmacy, and I was going to make an attempt to bring it.

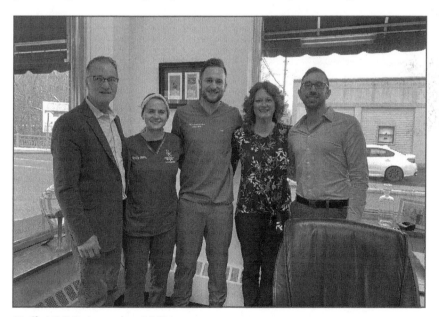

Staff at RC Outsourcing, LLC

◆ ◆ ◆

15
PUNISH THE LEGITIMATE
FOR NOT KNOWING
ONE FROM ANOTHER

T HE EVER-PRESENT SOCIAL BACKDROP to my business life was our nation's opioid addiction problem, and by 2015, the numbers were staggering. My brother-in-law, Judge John Durkin, had started one of the first drug courts in Ohio, served as president of the Ohio Judicial Conference, and was keeping me updated on the opioid problem. Reports of deaths and hospitalizations were constant, and the press seemed to have something to say about it daily. According to Judge Durkin, the average age of addicts fell from thirty-five to the early twenties, and heroin had replaced crack cocaine. Furthermore, prisons were disproportionately filling with people of color due to a racial bias; felony specifications based on previous arrest records made some eligible for the drug court option while excluding others. Our frequent conversations about the subtleties of the epidemic intrigued me and continued to drive my obsession with the law.

What had managed to stay below the radar in urban areas had now hit rural America, and tens of thousands were dying. That number would surpass hundreds of thousands in just a few years. Everyone was touched by this epidemic in some way or another, and it laid its ugly hand on the rich as well as the poor, the old and the young, brothers and sisters, and all occupations. The "just say no" strategy, with which we had been fighting the so-called War on Drugs since the 1980s, didn't envision a population that was just "following a doctor's orders" or a pharmacy profession that would print the orders on a label without being able to take the time necessary to decide if the drugs were for a legitimate medical purpose

Reading and comprehending the law as written and filtering out all the white noise created by the players who have distorted it over the years is not for the faint of heart, especially when looking to find parity between ideal and real. It's not possible to read the unadulterated laws and corresponding Board of Pharmacy rules and not see that something is wrong with pharmacy dispensing in the world of retail. Even if something didn't seem suspicious when contrasting the law against personal experience, hundreds of thousands of lives have been lost, and trillions of dollars of costs have been incurred, despite the laws meant to prevent such losses.

As dispensers of dangerous drugs—including Vicodin, Percocet, OxyContin, etc.—pharmacists have played a role in the development of a dangerous drug problem, especially since 75 percent of addictions began with prescriptions drugs. Until only recently, most of the blame has fallen on rogue physicians working "pill mill" clinics, wholesalers who were shipping too many bottles to pharmacies and should have known better, and manufacturers who should have known of the risk of addiction before marketing an FDA-evaluated and-approved drug. No one, oddly enough, was looking at the role of the pharmacist and the checks and balances they are legally required to provide. All the legal bloodhounds in this country chasing ambulances and malpractice claims, all the state and federal agencies, and even the people themselves failed to consider the one profession that was bound to watch out for and report the opioid addiction we are now witnessing.

Apparently, nothing about the way chain pharmacies filled prescriptions for dangerous drugs seemed inappropriate or reckless. Our experiences when visiting a pharmacy were so universal and commonplace that none of the activities we observed during the hustle and bustle of obtaining a prescription drug raised red flags because the public was unaware of OBRA-90 and had no basis to understand whether the law was being followed or not. And with the opioid epidemic now raging, every prescription filled at a pharmacy needed to be screened for legitimacy. The use of OBRA-90 laws needed to keep drugs out of the hands of those who had no medical reason to have them and do it in a way that was mindful of those who did. OBRA-90 was meant to prevent as much as it was meant to help.

As I had mentioned in an earlier chapter, I had an accident on a boogie board while on vacation and found myself in need of an opioid drug to treat my legitimate medical purpose, a broken neck. In the weeks following my accident, I had the unfortunate opportunity to experience the level of pain of someone who might later be unjustly stereotyped by the opioid epidemic. Legitimate patients who needed pain relief would be caught up in a frenzy of rule-writing meant to curb the activities of a profession that was unable to tell the needy from the abuser and so denied no one. Without being the cause of the opioid epidemic, legitimate pain patients would have to fight for their right to obtain relief.

When a pharmacist is pressured to fill a prescription in under a minute, it's impossible to tell a legitimate patient from someone who is about to pay their mortgage by reselling the drugs they just received. What should have been the labor-intensive dispensing process of asking twelve questions on the front end and discussing twenty-one drug facts during counseling was instead a sixty-second process that allowed abusers to walk in and walk out without catching the eye of the individuals who might have otherwise determined that they weren't taking these drugs at all.

Pharmacists weren't taking the time to ask why the patient was having a prescription filled. They weren't taking the time to read the notes entered by other pharmacists—if they had the time to enter them at all. And they weren't taking the time to perform a Drug Use Review, as the law requires. Since pharmacists weren't taking the time to counsel patients, as the law suggests, there was no time spent looking the patient in the eye to see if there were any red flags raised during the conversation, which would have led to more notes entered in the patient profiles.

The pharmacist who is simply typing up the exact instructions as written by a physician and placing the exact drug in a bottle as ordered is not considering the checks and balances established by law. Pharmacists do have a policing role to play, no matter how much pharmacy academia, corporate owners, and pharmacists themselves want to deny it. A rogue physician must not be allowed to operate undetected for an extended period, and dispensing laws clearly describe the pharmacist's expected role in preventing this.

Lawful dispensing practices police the use of dangerous drugs and also establish how legitimate patients can obtain them. By skirting OBRA-90 laws to maintain high prescription volumes, a pharmacist cannot tell an abuser from a legitimate pain patient, and those who need relief suffer when agencies drop the hammer on a distribution system that seems to be entirely illegitimate. The few are forced to bear the brunt of the deceptions perpetrated by the many, and the broad stroke that agencies took to "shut off the spigot" indicates that there was indeed broad violation of rules.

This lack of patient interaction, our inability to determine one type of patient from another, and the agency rules that followed can be taken a step further. Legitimate or not, these patients are human beings who became addicted at our hands, and just as it would be an injustice to suddenly discontinue pain management for legitimate patients, we should have stopped to consider the injustice we would do to abusers that we had illegitimately addicted.

In 2016, the CDC issued new guidelines that restricted the prescribing of opioids, and boards of pharmacy followed suit shortly thereafter by allowing limited quantities (14 days only) to be prescribed to "first-time" opioid users and setting prescribing standards for chronic use based on Morphine Milligram Equivalents" (MME). CVS Drug, our nation's largest pharmacy chain, did the same, as did other major chain pharmacies. And major drug wholesalers like Cardinal and Mckesson were limiting the number of bottles of opioids being shipped to retail pharmacies. This was creating shortages of pain medication on pharmacy shelves, jacking up prices, and forcing pharmacists to ration their dispensing.

This would have been fine if the drug being abused caused instant death and not addiction, but what about those already addicted? To whom could these citizens turn to satisfy the cravings our dispensing habits had fostered? Unable to turn to the legal pharmacy dispensers that just months before could guarantee an FDA-approved drug of exactly ten milligrams per dose, where would they go? Would their next dose come from a drug house and someone less scrupulous and be of unknown potency or purity? Pharmacy had played a role for years to foster addiction, and in a matter of just a couple of years would walk off the stage and take with them the source of relief for both legitimate and illegitimate patients.

Drugs like Fentanyl are measured in micrograms—one thousandth of a milligram. To create it, one must crush and evenly disperse the equivalent of a couple grains of sand throughout a bowl of inert powder. It cannot be done on a kitchen table inside a drug house with any measure of safety or reliability, yet this is the market we would force these patients to enter—legitimate and illegitimate alike—when agencies changed rules and corporate pharmacy backtracked from the opioid levels they were providing.

Had my neck not healed and my pain continued with the same intensity, I would have knocked on any door that promised relief. It's a level of pain one cannot understand without having felt it. Our misappreciation of spinal pain, coupled with our misunderstanding of addiction was all the ignorance of a biological process needed for the unfortunate loss of life that was to come.

At the risk of seeming too simplistic, addiction is memory, and our misguided notion that addiction is the desire to get high is what prevents us from understanding this strong evolutionary mechanism that drives addicts to seek the next dose. The high comes on first exposure, and although it can be felt again if the dosage is increased, what addicts are really seeking thereafter is relief from anxiety.

Humans have a defense mechanism that has developed over hundreds of thousands of years in which anxiety tells us where we can safely forage for food and where we must avoid. Imagine a distant human ancestor making its way toward a water source. It makes its way up a hill, around a large rock, over a log, and toward the water. When it reaches the watering hole, it is attacked by a predator, and with a burst of adrenalin released from an endocrine gland, it narrowly escapes to live another day. The short-term memory pathway established when the creature climbed the hill, walked around the rock, and jumped over the log are now bathed in adrenalin, creating fifty receptors along that pathway where once there were only five. The memory of the hill, the rock, and the log are now locked into long-term memory until a certain amount of time has passed—an amount of time dependent on the intensity of the event—or until that creature has nervously walked that same route again and again without incident. While our memory pathways print our maps, it's our anxieties that guide us as we follow them.

The brain receptors responsible for locking in memories, good or bad, need to be pinged with neurotransmitters like serotonin from time to time if they are to remain "alive" and steer our future movements away from danger or toward pleasure. The ratio between the number of receptors that need to be pinged and the amount of brain juice available to ping them determines our levels of anxiety. If an event is traumatic enough to create, say, five hundred receptors, like what was seen in "shell-shocked" patients in World War I, no amount of juice can be manufactured to satisfy them all, and the deficit can become so large that general motor functions are impaired. For most naturally occurring near-death experiences, however, it would not benefit a species if the number of receptors increased to a level that caused debilitation or for those receptors to stay active for a long period of time. Nature provides natural defenses to counter natural threats, so receptors are absorbed back into the nerve endings over time, the memory fades, and functioning calm can return. But like war, opioid consumption is not natural. And some, like fentanyl, are synthetic.

Opioids have the same effect on certain nerve endings as adrenalin and dopamine; the high that is felt when taking an opioid is like the high of adrenalin in that it creates fifty receptors that need to be pinged where there were only five before. This is why some American soldiers who fought in Vietnam reenlisted for combat duty even though they had just survived the hellish experience of jungle warfare. They had become addicted to an adrenalin high, and the receptors responsible for their anxiety could only be satisfied by this naturally occurring brain juice.

When these receptors are created naturally, if the individual can obtain the amount and type of sleep needed to replace exhausted stores of brain juice or receive intense counseling to convince them that the hill, rock, and log no longer pose a threat to them, the ratio between receptors and brain juice becomes manageable and their anxiety decreases. But this isn't the case with the opioid receptors of those who are addicted; only an opioid can satisfy the pings necessary, and no amount of sleep can manufacture enough chemicals to satisfy what is needed. Opioid receptors create unbearable amounts of anxiety when they aren't being doused with the drugs that opened them in the first place, and only with time can these receptors be reabsorbed. This can take months or even years, depending on the experience or the dose, which is why the insurance company practice of only paying for twenty-eight-day rehab stays should be reexamined.

Understanding this memory-based survival mechanism can help therapists appreciate the triggers that cause an addict to relapse. The memory of the top of the hill where the attack occurred is dramatic and can be calmed by tapping the air out of a syringe, holding a medication tablet, or receiving the dose itself, but it is only one of several "memories" that can serve as triggers if not considered as part of the entire initial experience. The rock has turned into a streetcorner that the individual frequented, and the log is a group of friends, a bar, or a drive in a particular car where drug residue remains in the ashtray. Those triggers associated with the addict's previous activities are difficult to avoid when the addict is eventually released from rehab. If the addict is without the financial means or familial support needed to return to the lush valley below the hill or shown a different watering hole from which to drink, they are destined to walk the same hill to drink from the only hole they know.

Downplaying the role of anxiety and the immense power it has to tell us where it's safe to walk and replacing it with an individual's selfish desire to get high is, in my mind, a simplistic view of the problem. Only pain moves someone to act with greater purpose than anxiety, and since unchecked anxiety will lead to the physical pain associated with flu-like symptoms, pain emerges as an additional driving force behind an addict's behavior. There is no desire for a high, no nasty upbringing, no misappreciation of the law that would cause a grandchild to put a gun to their grandmother's head to steal her money. Anxiety does that, and this kind of overwhelming, gut-shaking anxiety is childishly mistaken for wanting to get high.

Force yourself to stay awake for forty-eight hours, deplete your juice, tip the ratio in favor of the "normal" number of receptors you have, and see how you feel. Your skin will begin to itch, your muscles will spasm, and your nose might even begin to run because of the resources your body pulls from one area to another. If the depleted levels of brain juice are not restored, the normal receptors that are responsible for baseline thought processes begin to be absorbed back into nerve endings and become unavailable for things like coherent speech, memory, and joy. Brain function has now been permanently injured. This type of long-term damage was seen in dancers who participated in competitions in the 1920s and '30s to see who could stay on the dancefloor the longest. They suffered high rates of psychosis later in life, as did the radio announcers who tried to stay awake to cover the events.

Had I not been "blessed" with a self-limiting accident and my neck not healed as it had, I would have been one of the legitimate ones.

Instead, I needed only a single prescription to last me the couple of weeks it took for the swelling in my C-2 and C-3 vertebrae to go down. But if I had not been so fortunate, and the intense pain that I was feeling continued because major structural damage had occurred, I would have sought whatever relief necessary.

In such a miserably chronic state, it's only because of the fast pace set by chain pharmacies and their corporate-driven disregard of law that patients who are supposed to be seen as legitimately seeking pain relief would been seen as an abuser by a hurried chain pharmacist. Pharmacists are too busy to take the time to ask what happened, they stereotype need as abuse, and consequently make life difficult for those who already suffer. Patients seeking some measure of quality of life are tossed in with the abusers who ultimately were able to abuse because of the disregard dispensing pharmacists had for OBRA-90 and the protections it afforded legitimate pain patients.

Dispensing law violations created this problem, and pharmacists then lumped all patients together because they couldn't or wouldn't take the time to see people as individuals. Eventually, they would deny the addicted and the needy with such broad strokes of new agency rules and updated corporate chain policies that street venders replaced legal dispensers. Narcan, a prescription drug available only by prescription, could now be sold without a physician's orders. Legitimate pharmaceutical makers discovered that more money could be made with the increased sales of Narcan, administrators could stay busy instituting new rules and overseeing educational programs that explained its use, and chain pharmacists who would monitor distribution had yet another task to learn.

Pharmacists failed to see the addictive properties of OxyContin because they failed to see the patients who took it. The addictive properties of opioids are nothing new. The addictive nature of long-acting drugs over short acting is nothing new. OBRA-90 was nothing new, it just had not been used as the people intended, so we failed to catch what our profession already knew to be a possibility. We failed to look into the eyes of our patients, were not given enough time to document suspicions, and did as corporate emailed without having the means to resist their incentives or threats.

◆ ◆ ◆

16
THE REBIRTH OF A PHARMACISTS' ASSOCIATION

RC COMPOUNDING WAS OFFERED A CONTRACT with an insurance company, Pharmacy Benefit Manager (PBM), that would allow us to receive payment for prescriptions filled. My brother-in-law, the honorable Judge John Durkin from Mahoning County Court of Common Pleas, happened to walk into RC Compounding the day I was reading the contract, so I read him one of the clauses. The insurance company, in exchange for my receiving payment from them, would forbid me from "saying anything negative about the customer, the contract, physicians and nurses, or anyone else associated with the care of patients." His eyes widened and informed me that there might be something constitutionally wrong here.

Judge Durkin was my readily accessible go-to guy for the simple and sometimes not-so-simple questions I had when things like this popped up. I didn't always want to hear his careful reflections, but for the most part, I appreciated his willingness to steer me and my companies toward legal feasibility.

I didn't sign the contract. Here we were, in the grip of a national opioid epidemic, and an insurance company was telling me that I, as a dispenser of dangerous drugs, was not allowed to say anything negative. My own personal line in the sand had been crossed. This insult to the essence of OBRA laws and our "equal and corresponding responsibilities with physicians" could not be taken lying down. What pharmacies were signing these PBM contracts? Who was agreeing to this sort of stuff? Was this why pharmacists were forced to function like food-line robots, handing out drugs to citizens weren't speaking out? Were citizens only to be petted and patronized so more prescriptions could be dispensed per hour? Did this clause exist to prevent pharmacists from spending precious time confronting uncomfortable incidences of negative or abusive habits?

I was heading back into the world of professional pharmacy associations, but this time, with a newfound sense of urgency that wouldn't allow me to simply sit in on meetings that decided when best to meet again. I didn't want coffee and doughnuts and exchanges of business cards. I wanted organized activity, citizen petitions, and lawsuits. I decided to start by returning to my state association, OPA, to see if others felt the same outrage I did.

I had stayed away from the Ohio Pharmacists Association for several years, partially because I was embarrassed for the way I'd served as president, and partially because I had been busy growing my own businesses. I tried to maintain my membership, and now had a reason to want to sit on a committee. It was good to see some old friends when I traveled to Columbus to attend an OPA Membership Committee meeting. It was the first meeting I had attended in many years, and I hoped that chain pharmacy workplace conditions had reached a level that drew the notice it should. Sensing that it hadn't, I spoke with passion about finding a way to get these chain pharmacists off their asses—maybe even embarrass them, if need be—and confront the eight-hundred-pound gorilla that was filling one prescription per minute and ignoring OBRA-90 laws. We couldn't confront issues like "say nothing negative" if we continued to allow chain pharmacy to get away with creating and abiding by them.

We were losing independent pharmacies right and left, our college graduates were burning out in a matter of months, there was a shortage of jobs, and chain pharmacists were nowhere to be found except behind a pharmacy counter cranking out prescriptions at a dangerous rate, afraid to say anything negative. We were in the middle of our nation's costliest healthcare epidemic, with a healthcare system that had already spent trillions of debt-financed dollars, and we were wasting time going around the room discussing pleasantries. Committees were supposed to be the source of resolutions considered at our House of Delegates, yet nothing was happening, and each year only resolutions expressing appreciation to past officers were making it to the house floor.

When I was the OPA president, we argued openly and passionately at each spring's Annual House of Delegates meeting and then later in the evening enjoyed a beverage together. Now, we had all these issues that were causing serious problems for citizens, and no one wanted to speak freely—or, if they did, it was with the "political correctness" type of dialog that TV personalities would later make fun of.

One such issue that failed to garnish honest conversation became known as the "pain cream scam," and it involved compounding pharmacies. That same year, I sat on our OPA Compounding Committee and brought up this issue just as we were hearing about it. Pharmacists were inflating the price of the pain creams they were mixing for patients because insurance company computers had attached a high reimbursement rate to the raw ingredients used to make them. Compounding pharmacies were billing insurance companies $1,200 for a jar of cream that I, who didn't take insurance, sold for $30.

These pharmacies even sent representatives to physicians' offices soliciting prescriptions.

For our military alone, taxpayers were footing a bill of sometimes $15,000 a month for these particular concoctions. Prior to 2015, the Department of Defense paid very little for compounded drugs; just a year or two later, its total bill rose to over $300 million per month before their computers caught the offense.

I laid out the whole situation in a presentation to the committee, yet no one seemed to want to talk about it. Moral hazards were everywhere, even among compounding pharmacies. I knew compounders in my part of the state were partaking in this scheme, and while I was busy filling a few prescriptions per day, these other pharmacies only needed to fill a single prescription for one of these ridiculous creams to make it a good day at the office. This was an issue that should have skipped the "writing a resolution" stage and gone straight to "let's call a legislator."

Both OPA and APhA had a problem that perhaps no one could fix—not my friend Ernie Boyd at OPA nor Tom Menighan at APhA. They both led pharmacy organizations that had been created in the 1800s and structured to rely on pharmacists' participation to be effective. Instead of enjoying even modest levels of participation, they were fighting to hold the profession together against non-pharmacy entities like corporate administrators, insurance companies, and pharmacists themselves who were looking to tear it apart. And all the while, chain pharmacists sat on the sidelines, refused to join, said nothing in exchange for their high salaries, and accepted decrees restricting their freedom of speech.

Our associations were fighting without chain-pharmacy soldiers, all making fifty-to-sixty dollars an hour, none of them caring enough about what was going on around them to pay membership dues equal to a few hours of their work, and allowing corporate directives to erode the profession. The numbers who joined professional associations were pathetic; perhaps only one in fifteen chain pharmacists joined anything, and yet, they seemed to be causing nine out of ten problems that our profession faced. Even if they weren't directly causing the problems, they exacerbated them by turning their backs in apathy (or burnout) to those who were. Our associations were having to make bricks without straw, and I was very empathetic to this fact. But there was no way we could fight off the corporate wolves and protect our citizens from the abuse and misuse of prescription drugs without engaged members. It's that simple. And if pharmacists were afraid to say something controversial among their own peers, there was no way they were speaking out to their supervisors about working conditions or the inability to follow the law.

The professional laziness of the chain pharmacist had gone on long enough, and if they didn't come into the fold soon, I was going to embarrass them. I was going to call them out for what they were doing and the manner and the speed, in which they were doing it. I would bring this apathy and the skirting of the rules to the attention of the public. But first, I would try to gather together local pharmacists in a last-ditch effort and give them one more opportunity to speak out. They needed to be shown how democracy works, and I was going to do it by teaching them how to pass a resolution.

Back in the day, every county in our state had a local pharmacists' association. Pharmacists would get together once a month to have a couple of beers and talk about what was going on behind pharmacy counters in their districts. An OPA representative would travel from Columbus once a year to update our local association in Ohio and to keep the state organization abreast of local problems or concerns. They were local gatherings of like-minded individuals to redress our grievances. Yes, many individuals were competitors, but all that was put aside for the greater good of the profession and the public.

This level of association activity stopped when the demise of the independent pharmacy began to reduce the number of pharmacists who owned their own stores and felt a sense of community service. By 2012, most county pharmacy associations were either struggling or gone. The independent pharmacists who were personally connected with their communities had vanished, and all that remained were retail-chain pharmacists, and they didn't want to gather at all. Granted, we were losing this sense of community in most other industries as well, but ours involved dangerous drugs. Ironically, most independent pharmacists had a Bachelor of Pharmacy degree, while chain pharmacists, and all pharmacists, who graduated in 2000 or later were now required to hold a doctorate. One would think that the higher education requirement would have produced more civically minded individuals.

Nevertheless, I was going to give chain pharmacists the "benefit of the burnout" and reach out to them in the spirit of democracy. I was going to hunt them down and invite them personally, by email, or by phone to rejoin the process that could lead to solutions. Our local pharmacy association, called the Eastern Ohio Pharmacists Association, needed to fire back up and become involved in the decision-making process.

The Ohio Board of Pharmacy had always been accommodating when asked for a list of pharmacist names and addresses, and when I wanted to organize Eastern Ohio Pharmacists Association (EOPA), a new local association with six counties as members, Ohio's BOP was accommodating still. This time around, the data came in the form of an Excel spreadsheet that was emailed as an attachment. In the past, and when I requested a list of pharmacists in Ohio to solicit potential NAEP members, I was given hundreds of sheets of stickers with pharmacists' names and addresses on them to address envelopes.

Yay, I was no longer bound to snail mail! Although Yahoo limited the number of emails a person could send without raising the flag of spam, I got around this by sending as many emails as I could every twenty-four hours, day in and day out. Professional association life and the ability to send information was better now, especially since I had access to my own employees to help distribute notice of our organization's reactivation!

My typewriter had turned into a lightning-fast computer, and my ability to reach pharmacists with my words of encouragement and concern seemed boundless. I was my own boss who now owned two successful businesses, and I could say what I wanted without fear of a district supervisor walking in to scold me. All I needed to be wary of was my colleagues shunning me or a lawsuit from those I offended, so I tried to avoid both outcomes in my emails. I eventually contracted with a company that could send out all nine hundred emails at once with the push of a button, and my time was freed up to focus on what to say each Friday that might move my audience to action.

However, no movement would be complete without personal contact and physically passing out the type of information, that had once landed me in the unemployment line. Being self-employed, this was no longer a fear for me, so I hit the streets. My beat-up black Mercury Tracer had now turned into a shiny black Mercedes E-350, and in that, I started on Route 20 in Ashtabula County and worked westward, stopping at every pharmacy, clinic, and hospital I could find. Although MapQuest proved invaluable, there seemed to be a chain pharmacy at every intersection I came to, and after about a week, I managed to visit most all of them. The experience was exhilarating until my wife called me on my cell phone to ask where I was and what was I doing. Although I understood her concern, given all we'd been through because of my past professional association obsessions, I couldn't stop what I was doing, if for no other reason than the experience of it all.

Wearing a jacket and tie and carrying my clipboard, I probably looked a bit like Joann Predina. I suspect many pharmacists thought I was with the Ohio Board of Pharmacy because I never had to wait long at the pharmacy counter when I asked to speak with the pharmacist. I was never escorted out of the building for soliciting. Although a few pharmacists would quietly take my material and place it on the back counter out of the reach of store cameras, they returned to talk to me without drawing the attention of the out-front manager. These conversations were, again, absolutely exhilarating, and I think many of the pharmacists I talked to felt the same. A couple became teary-eyed when I talked about what our organization wanted to accomplish, while others offered a verbal litany of complaints they would like to see addressed. Only a few were standoffish, yet I would later see them at our meetings.

I traveled from Ashtabula County to Lake County, from Geauga to Trumbull, through Mahoning County, and on to Columbiana, seeing some old friends and making new ones. My personal visits, coupled with my deluge of emails, convinced me that we would have a good turnout for our first meeting. Membership applications kept the fax machine at RC Compounding busy, and it was not long before we surpassed six hundred members. We might have set a record for the largest local pharmacy association in the country.

Out top issue was democracy, not money, so we decided not to charge membership dues. I'm sure the "free meal" take on dues had something to do with our growth, but it was of no concern at the time. These chain pharmacists had finally been moved in a particular direction. EOPA was taking shape, and we had a body of members willing to listen. We could begin to institute change with the help of their guiding hands.

The officers of EOPA were appointed by divine decree, with heads on a desk and arms raised in the air. They consisted of old friends, past activists I knew, and one of my employees. We submitted our bylaws to the Ohio Secretary of State through an EOPA pharmacist and attorney, Carl Rafoth, esq. He had always been an active member of our local association in the past and was there for us again.

We set the date for our first EOPA meeting for October 15, 2013 and the number of RSVPs suggested that we would have a great turnout. The officers gathered to help prepare the paperwork that we would distribute at the meeting. We lined up speakers and ordered food and beverages. The theme of the meeting was both democracy and drug abuse, and we would gather in a ballroom in Niles, Ohio, the most central location within our district.

Joann Predina from the State Board of Pharmacy offered an hour of continuing education, and Antonio Ciaccia with OPA spoke about the issues pharmacy was confronting around the state. We invited Mahoning County Sheriff Jerry Greene to talk about the opioid abuse they were dealing with, and Judge Durkin spoke about the Mahoning County Drug Court he'd started and oversaw. News cameras from two TV stations were there, as were local newspaper reporters from the Youngstown Vindicator. Pharmacists also attended also—over 170 of them.

Our local pharmacy association had become one of the largest in the country and we were able to pull it together in a very short period. It was a testimonial to the fact that pharmacists (mostly retail) were finding themselves in a professional predicament where they had not been before. Most of the pharmacists in attendance were chain pharmacists. They were beginning to feel the job market closing in on them, and the jobs they did have were growing increasingly frustrating.

EOPA had a great start and we began in earnest to plan our next meeting.

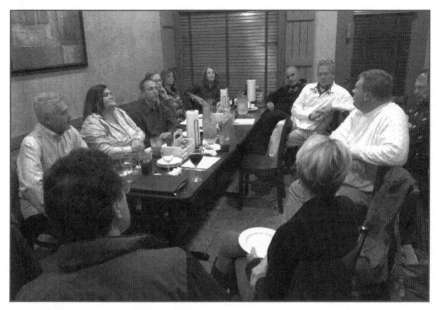

EOPA Officers meet to discuss pharmacy issues

◆ ◆ ◆

17

Testing the Waters
with Resolution and Law

E OPA's second meeting was held on April 24, 2014. It focused on professional representation and why most issues in our field were the direct result of our lack of it. Senator Joe Schiavoni was our guest speaker, and later he would make the comment on a radio talk show that he felt as though the "crowd" was agitated about something and felt like they wanted to take out their frustrations on him. Joe Sabino, R.Ph.and long-time OPA treasurer and friend provided an hour of continuing education. The meeting was well attended, we swore in our new officers, established a board representative from each county, and passed a resolution asking that the next executive director to be selected later that year be required to be a pharmacist.

I provided a PowerPoint that highlighted the number of pharmacists in our state and country and contrasted this with the dismal number who were members of professional organizations. I explained why it's important for an individual experience behind the pharmacy counter to be shared with others to determine if they had the same experience and if it was of concern. If it was, local officers could then bring that concern to the state organization. Maybe something happening in a town was also happening around the state, and maybe it was something of importance.

I was particularly concerned about the "say nothing negative" clause in PBM's contract and felt that every pharmacist should view it as the ultimate insult. This wasn't what our members believed was most important, however, and we knew that in advance of the meeting. We used Survey Monkey to ask our 650 members what their greatest concern was, and we put the top result in a written resolution for them to debate and vote on. Our members' greatest concern: they wanted a *lunch break*.

I explained the resolution's wording and the written fix. Then, there was a thoughtful debate and a vote of the membership present. Without this structure and calculated directives coming from the membership, what are officers supposed to forward to legislators, oversight agencies, or maybe even employers? Change must come from an organization's membership, not the organization's leader; otherwise, it's just the leader's thoughts. Without membership, there is no broad consensus, and without that, no one can guarantee that a potential solution to a problem will be in the best interests of the majority. No solution thought up and forwarded by one officer can hope to be as all-encompassing or impactful as those derived from and supported by a quorum of individuals. Membership gives weight and hopefully the financial resources necessary to put a solution into practice. Everything else is lobbyist-driven returns on investment.

We had a championship lineup of players—if only those players decided to get into the game. Although I didn't want to scold those in attendance, I didn't want to patronize them, either. The data was the data, and they would either accept it or not. I felt very confident that I had portrayed this issue of pharmacist apathy as the source of all our problems. Now, I just had to see if they accepted this message.

We presented our "Lunch Break Resolution" for the meeting attendees' consideration, the membership debated it, and it passed. Although the process didn't need to use Robert's Rules of Order, it was still a hard-fought victory for pharmacy democracy in northeastern Ohio and rang out with an angelic tone of "Yeas" in the harmony one would expect of like-minded individuals joining together for a purpose.

We advanced our EOPA resolution to OPA's annual meeting held later that spring in Columbus. There, it was debated, voted on, and rejected because it smelled of mandates and many were opposed to any rule that would force an employer to have to do something. While I'm not in favor of mandates, asking for a lunch break—which chain pharmacists were asking for—could have made for a nice olive branch to draw more chain pharmacists into our state association's fold.

This rebirth of our local association didn't garner much OPA or APhA press, and chain pharmacist membership didn't increase in either association despite our pleas locally to join. Since the main theme of our first meeting was the opioid epidemic, and we were combining the role of the pharmacist with it, both our state and national pharmacy associations remained silent on our activities. Both associations still failed to see the long-term benefit they stood to gain by helping us foster the message that membership was the number-one issue and that all other issues we faced could be resolved if we remained focused on this most important of professional deficits. Instead, they spit out the cure because one symptom of our apathy tasted bitter to them.

Following our disappointment at the state level, EOPA entered a period of calm. It quickly became apparent that we needed to sustain an intense effort to keep chain pharmacists' interest in participating. There was no way around it: these chain pharmacists wanted free food, free continuing education and face-painting, or they weren't going to attend. Despite our accomplishment of gathering so many pharmacists in one room, the same few who already consistently gathered would be the few who would continue to show up at future meetings. There were no donations, no emails, no social media comments or likes, and no input from the chain-pharmacy sector section. It was a frustrating battle to fight.

A meeting we would later host at a beautiful winery in Ashtabula had but five attendees, including myself and one of my students from ONU, and this made me more angry than embarrassed. Another event that we hosted on a beautiful sunny day for Ohio gubernatorial candidate Senator Schiavoni was also sparsely attended. It was held in an outside pavilion where we had catered food, free beverages, and a chance to talk one-on-one with a leader who had often gone to bat for us on the radio and TV. My wife joked that half of those who attended were members of our family and not members of EOPA. It wasn't the wasted food that agitated me but the fact that we had come so close to delivering a message about working conditions that could have made a difference, had our membership taken it and run.

My high had hit a low, and so, I begin attacking pharmacists more frequently on social media and in the news. I was still in their corner, but overdose deaths were hitting every corner of the map, and there was no way this profession could escape having hard conversations about cause and effect. I wasn't blaming the individual pharmacist for causing this epidemic, but I knew our role in drug distribution was important, and I began to focus more on dispensing laws. This lawful pivot brought me closer to the public, and I felt more comfortable talking to them about these issues than a room of pharmacists. I was tired of arguing with professional associations on social media about why they weren't having conversations about opioid use and workplace conditions. My conversations with family and friends about what a pharmacist should be doing were more reassuring than those I was having with fellow pharmacists. I heard too many pharmacists argue some version of "everyone practices this way, so it must be correct."

EOPA wasn't done, but my feelings about pharmacists' apathy had moved me into the public's corner, and there I would stay. I was beginning to look for the same safety in numbers that I was encouraging pharmacists to find when addressing workplace conditions. I began to think that maybe we needed an educated public to force chain pharmacies to address conditions. To accomplish this, however, I would need to find the right amount of embarrassment to lay at the feet of pharmacists without tripping over it myself. But how could I inform the public about dispensing laws? And would they be a good judge of lawful intent if they heard it? I needed to gather lawyers and citizens together and "run it up the flagpole" to know for sure.

The lobby of the old bank building where RC Outsourcing is located was the perfect venue for such a gathering. It was an open space with a good view of the restored vault where physical wealth had once been stored. The walls were adorned with portraits and lithographs of past presidents, and centered above these was a large painting depicting the signing of the Declaration of Independence. The space reeked of the type of democracy that had protected our citizens while affording them wealth, and it was the ideal place to test my understanding that pharmacists had a role to play in the opioid epidemic.

I called the gathering the RC Legal Forum and I hosted it in March of 2016.

I invited Mahoning County Coroner Dr. Joseph Ohr to speak about what he was seeing postmortem in opioid overdose deaths. His explanation of the "foam cone" that comes out of an overdose victim's mouth as they gasp for their last breath was very moving. Judge Durkin from the Mahoning County Drug Court talked about the types of drugs he was seeing abused and the resulting life and property loss. Then, in front of pharmacists, lawyers, and a judge, I gave a PowerPoint presentation on federal OBRA laws, corresponding Ohio Board of Pharmacy rules, and my own explanation of what was expected under each. The question I posed that evening was whether all these elements of dispensing could be done in under sixty seconds, and I provided many visual examples of why we should consider that an impossibility.

TV cameras were rolling when I asked the question of how it was possible that we never knew just how addictive OxyContin was, when everything written in the law was meant to expose and prevent it. OBRA-90's Drug Use Review begins with the words "In order to thwart the abuse and misuse of prescription drugs . . ." Did the public even know that such a law existed and that it had been passed in 1990, long before our citizens' addiction to opioids began? The data shows that 75 percent of addictions began with prescription pain pills, yet no one was looking at a law that was enacted to thwart abuse and misuse.

Physicians were being arrested and given jail sentences. Wholesalers and drug manufacturers were being sued. And yet, no one was looking at the "trusted pharmacist," bound to laws necessary to control drug distribution, as a target for change. Chain-retail pharmacists were too apathetic to join an organization and speak out about the conditions they faced, too frightened of losing their high-paying jobs, and yet content enough to lock the gates at night, hoping that no one would put together a PowerPoint explaining it all. But I put one together and delivered it that evening. No one disagreed with my analysis or offered any point of contention. This was the confirmation that I was looking for. I needed to continue working hand-in-hand with the people to right this wrong. For the first time that I know of, the public had an opportunity to learn about drug dispensing laws and the legal community was given the opportunity to consider their relevance to our opioid epidemic and the importance of the profession of pharmacy for the checks and balances described in them.

This RC Legal Forum aired on local TV stations and was covered in the local papers. Not surprisingly, neither OPA nor APhA gave the event any press, nor did they mention it on social media. I understand that the subject probably seemed embarrassing to the profession and perhaps to the leaders of our associations, whose job was to promote the profession, not degrade or speak ill of it. I, however, felt that protecting the profession was just as important as promoting it, and I'm sure that responsibility can be found somewhere in their bylaws. Despite the silent condemnation, I was firmly focused on the role of corporate owners holding my colleagues' reins, and that is who I was implicating, not individual pharmacists.

The profession needs to be protected by ensuring that the laws and rules that define us are being upheld and practiced; if they aren't, we will cease to exist. Our situation was everyone's and no one's fault. Perhaps it was even the public's fault for their desire for discounts and speed.

Either way, our drug misuse issues were of such a grave nature that we had no time to point fingers and very little time to acknowledge where we had strayed and get back on course before the people knocked us there. This quote by Thomas Jefferson says it best: "If our house be on fire, without inquiring whether it was fired from within or without, we must try to extinguish it."

I would remain at a slow simmer while I jumped into another project that would keep me busy and keep my mind off the professional cold shoulder I had received. Our Legal Forum confirmed that

I was correct in my understanding of the law and that we needed to use the law to pull us back. How practical that was given the extent to which our profession had drifted, the number of players involved, and the amount of money being made was another matter.

My interview at the end of the evening was the first time a reporter had expressed concern for my personal safety. I knew that I was talking about a subject that many others in various positions within pharmacy would not want to hear, accept, or want published. Major chain pharmacies were making billions of dollars in profit, administrators and academia enjoyed employment in this world of status quo, and agencies might not have appreciated that I was suggesting that they were failing to do their jobs. Be that as it may, I knew that my topic was the sort of stuff movies were made of, and many times there fails to be a happy ending for the instigator.

Personally, I didn't enjoy the fact that I had just hung myself out on TV, and that night I was made aware that I'd done so by the cameraman who covered the event. I was not a whistleblower who stood to collect a certain percent of monies for my words, and my businesses stood to gain nothing from my pharmacy activism. And although there were times when I found myself to be a bit more cautious than usual, I never experienced a threat. I tried to discount the notion that drug manufacturers, chain pharmacies, and insurance companies were powerful entities with all the ability in the world to silence me. I was too far along in my efforts and was not the type to stop here. The evening had given me a validation based in law, OBRA-90, and this law belongs to the people. I felt more comfortable being with them than I did in the company of my colleagues who offered silent disregard.

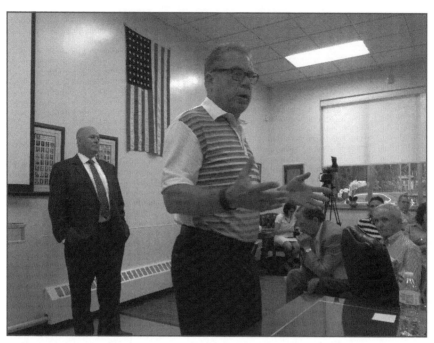

Honorable Judge John M. Durkin speaks at RC Legal Forum with County Coroner Dr. Joseph Ohr in the background.

◆ ◆ ◆

18
POSSIBLE UNEMPLOYMENT
AWAKENS THE DEAD

AROUND THIS TIME IN 2016, I was beginning to make regular appearances on the *Louie B. Free Show*. Louie is a 1960s-era hippie with all the compassion for others that you might expect from someone like him. His utopian view of the world and its problems are displayed weekly in the myriad of famous and not-so-famous guests he has on his show.

One day, I received a call from a pharmacist friend who told me that this guy wanted to talk to me, so I called him. Louie wanted to know if I would be willing to come on his show to talk about anything I wanted to talk about. I felt as though I might have some interesting topics to discuss, so I said yes. Little did I know that I was about to forge one of my most cherished friendships.

Louie and I hit it off in that first show we did together, and I was able to get a little airtime to talk about different subjects that were dear to me. He also has a large Facebook following, which we linked together as Facebook friends, and between his social media influence and our radio sessions, I was able to share my message and activities with a larger audience. Also, I liked knowing that my message was being recorded.

The opioid epidemic was by now in full swing, and passions were running high everywhere. But the pharmacy issue that would once again bring our local association together was a report that chain pharmacies were about to try out a dispensing system that would allow a pharmacy technician to sign off on another pharmacy technician's work before handing the drug to the patient. "No pharmacist necessary" was exactly the kind of juicy subject that I needed to share with EOPA members in my Friday newsletters.

Having set off alarms about possible pharmacists' unemployment, we were soon receiving email feedback suggesting that we had struck an important nerve. These pharmacists seemed ready and willing to meet again, and the part of me that had sought to buddy up with the public found their eagerness amusing. Here they were, ready to meet in order to fend off the unemployment that their unwillingness to meet had created. Their poor working conditions and potential unemployment were only symptoms of their apathy and unwillingness to band together.

This report came from the National Association of Chain Drug Stores (NACDS), and although their name might sound as though they offer professional representation to chain pharmacists, they don't. A member had to own five or more stores, and annual dues were determined by the annual sales of the chain. Individual chain pharmacists are unable to join, elect officers, or hold office themselves, and the organization's agenda was determined by the owners and/or representatives of various chain pharmacies.

It's difficult to know for sure how much lobbying money a Walmart, CVS, or Walgreens could contribute to further the organization's agenda, but I imagine it's a sizable amount. Without a chain pharmacists' association to counter their efforts, there would be very little pushback against their activities unless a state or national pharmacy association that represents all pharmacists was willing to forgo their chain relationships to provide it. Of late, we are seeing more state and national pharmacy associations taking a stand against chain pharmacies due to the workplace conditions they have created.

I didn't visit any stores to promote EOPA's next meeting; I just continued sending out Friday morning emails. Everyone is in a good mood on Fridays, so I figured people would be more likely to take the time to read my messages. Attached to the newsletter was the resolution that we would debate and vote on at our spring EOPA meeting. It simply said that given what we saw happening behind pharmacy counters and what the law said should be happening, we would petition government agencies, namely our Ohio Board of Pharmacy, to investigate whether dispensing rules were being followed. It was everything I thought we would need to send a letter to the Ohio Board of Pharmacy. I hoped that a message sent on behalf of such a large organization might get their attention enough to look at how prescriptions were being filled in under sixty seconds.

My message to the EOPA members read:

March 16, 2017

Dear Fellow Pharmacists,

EOPA officers and staff met tonight to ready your packets for this Sunday night's meeting in Niles. Please see the invite . . . we think we have an enjoyable program for you!

While stuffing packets, we concluded that many might not know what our resolution means . . .

The representatives of the chain industry (NACDS) are involved in a pilot program to test whether certain responsibilities of a pharmacist could be done as competently by one technician checking another. While we understand the need to expand our

clinical skills and lessen the burdens of volume, our resolution (our group) will ask for an assessment of current pharmacy practice and whether these «business models» continue us on the same path we have been seeing over the past 20 yrs. or so. **It is neither pro nor con Tech-check-Tech but speaks to our defined responsibilities (education)**

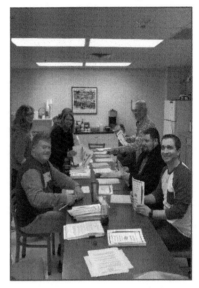

as pharmacists and the conversation that needs to happen before being further removed from them. *As important as it is to expand our clinical functions, the people of Ohio have specific laws and rules in place that require us to be certain we know who is receiving a prescription and the appropriateness/ legitimacy of it. The trend of moving from prospective (DUR/ Profiling) to retrospective (MTM) to accommodate volume needs to be addressed.*

Please see the attached Resolution. *It can be passed as is, amended/changed, or rejected completely.* **This will be up to those present to decide when we vote.** *If the group feels we have talked too long about it, someone can move to end debate and voting would take place at that time. This is an open mic and all are free to speak.*

The doors open at 6:00PM. **Please come and support us.**

The EOPA spring meeting fell on my birthday, March 19, 2017, and I was hoping for a present in the form of a resolution. Attendance was good, and adrenaline was high. It was an election year (primary) so everyone running for legislature wanted time to speak. Ernie Boyd from OPA was there, as were TV cameras and newspaper reporters. I visited with pharmacists at their tables before the meeting to give one last push to get our resolution passed. It centered on workplace conditions and the high volumes of prescriptions being filled, and slipped into the mix was the notion that we had rules to follow that weren't being followed. For good measure, it also asked that colleges and professional associations reexamine their priorities, end their silence, and come to the aid of chain pharmacists.

EASTERN OHIO PHARMACISTS ASSOCIATION

March 19, 2017
A Resolution
Tech—check—Tech

Whereas the National Association of Chain Drug Stores has partnered with the Pharmacy Society of Wisconsin to pilot a new practice model based on prescription verification involving technicians only;

Whereas current Ohio law and Board of Pharmacy rules do not recognize such practices;

Whereas pharmacists need relief from high prescription volume environments in addition to assistance from highly trained technicians;

Resolved, that the *Eastern Ohio Pharmacists Association*:

1. Urges the officers of EOPA and the Ohio Pharmacists Association to engage in conversation with organizations and agencies to ensure public safety is held paramount.

2. Asks academia and professional associations to re-evaluate the responsibilities of pharmacist dispensing functions according to the Ohio Administrative Code.

3. Requests that agencies examine current dispensing practices and assess the potential impact it has had on drug distribution prior to enacting any new law or rule that will further separate pharmacists from their lawful duties and responsibilities.

When the resolution was introduced, I gave a quick speech about what it meant. It passed unanimously without debate, and I received my birthday present. The meeting was a success in that we'd obtained a consensus from a large group of pharmacists who put into writing a call for action. EOPA could now send a letter to our Ohio BOP asking for their consideration.

The next day, the local TV news coverage in the *Vindicator* began: "The Local Pharmacists association took action tonight by passing a resolution asking the state board of pharmacy to be stricter." As with previous meetings, our meeting's official theme was opioid addiction. It was the second publicly televised event in which we made the connection between potential rule violations happening behind pharmacy counters and our nation's opioid-abuse problem.

Pharmacists meeting in Niles discuss opioid epidemic

The opioid epidemic sweeping the nation was one of the topics discussed by members of the Eastern Ohio Pharmacists Association this past weekend.
Monday, March 20th 2017, 12:18 AM EDT
Updated: *Sunday, April 2nd 2017, 5:23 PM EDT*

The opioid epidemic sweeping the nation was one of the topics discussed by members of the Eastern Ohio Pharmacists Association this past weekend.

Ohio Senator Joe Schiavoni (D) was there asking the group of 200 pharmacists about some of the issues they may experience in the workplace.

"I sensed a lot of frustration from them. They are just trying to serve people and help people and they want to be able to have that human interaction with their patients and when you hammer them with a bunch of different requirements. It's hard to do that," said Senator Schiavoni.

In Ohio, there is no law mandating the amount of breaks pharmacists can take during a shift or the maximum amount of prescriptions they can fill in an hour.

In Illinois, a bill is pending that considers these factors. Senator Schiavoni discussed with the group if that's something Ohio needs to consider.

"I wanted to come and actually talk to the pharmacists and I think they do have some pressures. I don't know if they are willing to say they need to unionize or they are willing to say we need this legislation in order to survive. It seems like more of the problems were coming from the pricing and dealing with the cost and distribution and the explanation to the patients," Senator Schiavoni said.

Ray Carlson of the Pharmacists Association told 21 News, the opioid addiction rate is the biggest problem and they are urging the state consider the legislation.

"Seventy-five percent of heroin overdoses began with prescription pain medication and we feel that pharmacists are a key component of the drug distribution," said Carlson.

After I completed my TV interview at the meeting and the camera was turned off, the reporter asked me if I was afraid that someone might put a bomb under my car. It was the second time a reporter had suggested that my personal safety may be at risk for pursuing this issue, but I didn't think much of it at the time. Only later, when my democratic process progressed into a courtroom, would that question lodge deeper in my psyche.

When I had suggested to EOPA officers that pharmacists shared some responsibility for the opioid epidemic, some were taken aback. According to many of my pharmacist colleagues, the blame rested squarely on the shoulders of the physicians who were writing the prescriptions and the pharmacist's only responsibility was to ensure that the information on a prescription vial was exactly as the physician had written it and that the bottle contained the correct pills ordered by the physician. The claim that we were responsible for doing more than that put pharmacists and the profession in a bad light and wouldn't be popular in pharmacy circles. I was very sensitive to the "it's not my fault" attitude, and I tried to reassure them that we were talking about and blaming corporate-owned pharmacies and their business models, not individual pharmacists.

The day following our EOPA meeting, I drafted a letter to our Board of Pharmacy and notified our officers that it only awaited their signatures. By day's end, it was clear that half had no intention of signing. Those who refused were working for retail-chain pharmacies, and they feared retribution.

I had worked in retail-chain pharmacies for years, and I knew exactly how they felt; to be quite honest, if I were still in their shoes, I probably wouldn't have signed the letter, either. I too had a family to provide for, and in Ohio, as in most other states, employment is "at will." That means that under Ohio law, an employee is generally free to quit their job for any reason. On the other hand, an employer can generally terminate an employee for any reason—or even for no reason at all—so long as the reason doesn't violate the law. I probably knew this better than those officers who were unwilling to sign the letter and I understood their position, even though I still pushed for their signatures. We were just officers acting on behalf of a membership. We were just the messengers, and yet, even messengers can be fired for "no reason" in Ohio.

In the end, the EOPA letter describing the action we wanted the Board of Pharmacy to take was never sent, and our resolution was not considered at the spring OPA House of Delegates meeting since it wasn't received by the Resolutions Committee on time. Just as I suspected, our resolution garnered no association press and no social media coverage.

I was done arguing with pharmacists and pharmacy administrators. I was now going to speak entirely to and on behalf of the public. The apathy, reluctance, and cold shoulder I had received from my own colleagues and pharmacy associations had drawn my line in the sand for me. All I could do now was hope that a similar apathy didn't exist among the public.

Something was bouncing around in the minds of these chain pharmacists that caused their reluctance to participate and speak out against their employers, and it was something I was all too familiar with. At the end of a busy day filling prescriptions, when all they wanted to do was escape their reality and pretend things weren't so bad, who would want to worry about potential conflict with an employer? This speaks to their innocence, despite all their civic education and social responsibilities.

The reluctance to challenge an abuser and pretend that life will get better is a real phenomenon that society is all too familiar with. There are times when it's just not possible to run from an abusive relationship, to call the authorities, or to ask loved ones for help. Sometimes, there are children involved. Sometimes, the abused depends on the abuser's income. And so, the abused will wait, hoping that others who are in a position to notice the offense will intervene and put a stop to it without threatening their physical or financial well-being.

In 2017, intervention and safety were not coming to chain pharmacists, though, so they kept their heads down and tolerated their employers' abuse as best they could. Eventually, seeing that abuse was all around them in every chain they might escape to, chain pharmacists decided that this was just the new normal of pharmacy that they would have to survive. The need to "dumb-down" their existence was the only way to survive a level of abuse that even the "thinkers" within the industry failed to challenge. Who would be the first victim of abuse to claim that what was happening to them was wrong, when agencies, academia, and associations themselves were turning their backs on the suggestion?

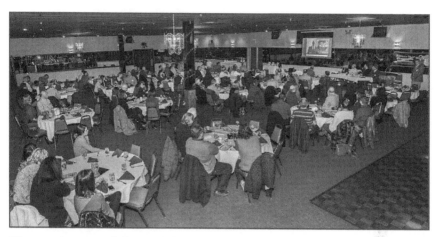

Pharmacists attend EOPA meeting to consider a resolution

❖   ❖   ❖

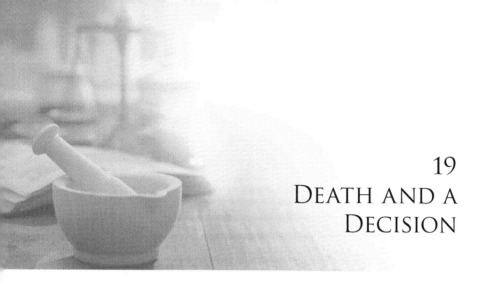

19
DEATH AND A
DECISION

ONE WEEK BEFORE OUR MARCH, 2017 EOPA MEETING, a friend
of mine drove past RCO as I was taking out the trash. He rolled down
his window and asked if he and his wife could make an appointment
to see me so I could go over her prescriptions and help them make
some sense of what she was taking. I don't take appointments for
medication counseling, and certainly not for close friends, but I told
him that he could stop in anytime during business hours.

This friend was an ex-Marine who had rappelled onto the roof
of the US embassy in Beirut, Lebanon, after it was bombed in 1983.
He and his wife were very close, and they rode through most of
the continental United States together on his motorcycle for their
honeymoon. She had diabetes and fibromyalgia, was taking a lot of
prescription medications from several different physicians, and was
having them all filled at a local chain pharmacy. Her maintenance
medications, those that were being taken chronically, were being
filled by a mail-order pharmacy.

Five days after our EOPA meeting, my friend's wife was found
dead on their living room couch. She was forty-nine years old. The

paramedics were unable to resuscitate her, and their blood glucose monitor showed the possible reason why. Her blood sugar had fallen so low that she fainted before she could call for help, and it continued to fall until she eventually passed away.

After her funeral, I asked my friend to bring me her prescription bottles so I could see whether there might have been some connection between her death and the medications she was taking. I was shocked by the number of medications and OTC supplements she was taking, but also by the way her medications were arranged in her plastic daily pill reminder pack. It was obvious that both were clueless about what needed to be taken and when. They had doubled up her doses of some, skipped others, and had received four different prescriptions from two different physicians that essentially combined two of the same medications. She was taking nearly seventeen medications and supplements and had an implanted insulin pump to regulate her blood sugar. It was obvious that no one had explained anything to her about the drugs she was taking.

She had died about two weeks after receiving a prescription for twenty milligrams of Prednisone to be taken three times a day. The prescription was written for 270 tablets, with three refills, but she was able to handle only a couple weeks of it before her sugar crashed. She was never warned that her blood-sugar levels could be affected by the steroid, nor told about any potential side effect, adverse reactions, what to do if she missed a dose, how to store it, or when to take it. These instructions were simply printed in small font and stapled to the bags.

I asked my friend if anyone behind the pharmacy counter had asked if she had a medical device like an insulin pump. "No," he said. "They just asked for a birthdate and a phone number" so they could find her in the computer.

Then, I asked my friend if they had ever talked to a pharmacist. He said, "No. They asked us if we had any questions, but what the hell did we know to ask?" Not once had a pharmacist come out from behind the counter to tell them anything about the drugs she was taking. The only time they ever talked to someone at the pharmacy was when the pharmacy staff called to say that a refill prescription was on its way, and they seemed to get such a call every other day. They weren't even calling to have the prescriptions refilled; they were just coming on auto-fill. My friend and his wife had been filling their prescriptions at the local independent pharmacy until their insurance notified them that they had to transfer to a chain pharmacy and use mail-order for maintenance medications.

Chain pharmacies and mail-order pharmacies face many of the same problems. Both must carry a Terminal Distributor License, and the rules governing them are the same. But while one pharmacist at a chain pharmacy averages sixty prescriptions an hour, a mail-order pharmacist can average two hundred. Crucially, we are unable to peer inside the workings of mail-order facilities because we're separated from them by a 1-800 number. The category of professionalism is the same at both, and they can be thought of as one category of pharmacy workplace, since they're often owned by the same corporations and investors. Both were dispensing medications to my friend's wife.

The loss of this beautiful person at age forty-nine hit many of us hard. I was especially upset, knowing what I did about patient safety and the laws necessary to ensure it. I had spent many years trying to address exactly what my friend had hoped I could help him with. This man was the skilled carpenter who finished the wood trim inside our new federal courthouse building and built doors for our beloved Butler Museum of Art in Youngstown, yet he would not know justice. He had to declare bankruptcy because of the money he owed to a health-care industry that had possibly contributed to his wife's death. It's an all-too-common story. The assault on an individual is sometimes too complicated, too vague, and too far away from the perpetrators to find relief before the one-year statute of limitations expired.

I made up my mind to no longer argue about irresponsible dispensing practices with fellow pharmacists and the pharmacy associations who were supposed to represent them. Instead, I was going to circulate a citizen's petition and deliver it personally, along with our local association's resolution, to our Board of Pharmacy in Columbus. I was going to bring this issue to the attention of the public and act on their behalf as best I could. I was going out on that proverbial "limb" of my profession, and my last hope was that the people wouldn't leave me hanging there once they understood what was at stake. It was a complicated issue that would require their understanding, and I would do my best over the next few years to explain it. I was worried but not afraid. I had cash now and could hire any lawyer I wanted, but ultimately, I would need the public to see past the confusion and understand the importance of this issue enough to want to do something about it.

Immediately following the death of my friend's wife, I drafted a citizen's petition and began to circulate it for signatures. It read:

TO PETITION THE OHIO BOARD OF PHARMACY TO EXAMINE CURRENT DISPENSING PRACTICES

Raymond Carlson, RPh Ohio 22 Comments
(ONLY FOR RESIDENTS OF OHIO)

We, the undersigned, are concerned citizens of Ohio who urge our Board of Pharmacy to examine various levels of compliance with OBRA-90, ORC and OAC as related to:

pharmacist counseling, prospective drug utilization review, pharmacist-specific notations (prospectively) in patient profiles that are relevant to individual drug therapies, *the levels of compliance obtained through automation verses thoughtful pharmacist interaction*, and conclude whether or not these occurrences satisfy the intended meaning of Ohio law as established by the people in order to thwart abuse and misuse of prescription medications.

According to Ohio law, pharmacists share equal and corresponding responsibility with physicians to ensure that a prescription is written for a legitimate medical purpose. In consideration of Ohio's opioid addiction rate and deaths due to overdose, hospitalizations due to preventable medication errors, a voluntary Ohio Drug Take-Back program that nets 18 tons of unused drugs in 2016, investigative reports in other states, the growth of MTM (retrospective), studies which show 90% over-ride rates on DUR warnings, high rate (90%) of patient counseling declines evidenced in log books, and the absence of voluntary error reporting; *we ask the Ohio Board of Pharmacy to determine whether or not there is reasonable pharmacist compliance with OAC rules and standards of care in retail outpatient and mail-order pharmacies that either reside or do business within our state.* The standards of care in this petition are especially but not limited to:

OAC 4729-5-18

OAC 4729-5-20

OAC 4729-5-21

OAC 4729-5-22

Once I had received a couple hundred signatures, I added this petition to our EOPA Resolution and various stories in the press about the dangers of hurried workplace conditions in pharmacies. Then, I bundled it all together and made the trip to Columbus to deliver it to the Ohio Board of Pharmacy in person.

As I sat in the waiting room, I noticed the BOP's mission statement hanging on the wall above me, which read:

Mission Statement

The State of Ohio Board of Pharmacy shall act efficiently, consistently, and impartially in the public interest to pursue optimal standards of practice through communication, education, legislation, licensing, and enforcement.

It was the "enforcement" part of the statement and the recent death of my friend's wife that gave me the much-needed courage to walk in and tell the Board exactly what I thought needed to be enforced. I explained why I thought inspectors needed to visit retail-chain pharmacies and look at patient profiles, see how many prescriptions were being filled per hour, and flip through the pages of counseling logs to see how many patients were declining this important service. I thought the meeting went well, and their staff was very professional, so when I returned to Lowellville, I filled out an application to have my petition added to the agenda of the next Board of Pharmacy meeting. The application was received, and the issue would be considered at their July meeting.

That summer, I drove to Columbus for the BOP meeting. I made my way up to the conference room where the meeting was being held. I signed in on the attendance sheet next to the many chain pharmacy industry representatives who regularly attended and took my seat to wait for my item on the agenda to be called.

The board members must not have received the petition in advance, so they were given a few minutes to read it. I expected that there wouldn't be much conversation about it, and there wasn't. I could empathize with Executive Director Steve W. Schierholt, Esq., when he shook his head slightly and muttered something about not knowing how something like this could be accomplished. After all, I wasn't making claims about specific dispensing violations; I was arguing that the entire chain industry was violating dispensing rules. This was a huge accusation involving many licensed facilities operated by many licensed individuals. Only one board member spoke in favor of giving the petition further consideration, and since I wasn't allowed to address the board due to time constraints that they had announced at the beginning of the meeting, it failed for lack of evidence or interest. My petition received a couple of sentences in the board's minutes, and that was that.

Our BOP was already severely underfunded and understaffed to effectively combat the never-ending problems faced by pharmacists, and now, our state legislature was expecting them to also develop and oversee the legal distribution of medical marijuana. I understood all this and spoke frequently on-air about the difficulties our BOP faced. Still, I was frustrated that they wouldn't even let me say a few words after they tabled my petition. I would wait out six months of BOP inactivity before deciding to file a lawsuit against them.

The machinery of governmental agencies and professional associations was too slow for my level of patience. Everyone knew the number of opioid deaths happening around us and the number of families being affected. Those numbers represented the deaths of citizens like my friend's wife, but the uncounted and unrecognized loss of life was too vague and without enough compelling evidence to trace an incident back to a single culprit. Had these agencies viewed these distant deaths with the same clarity that the New England Compounding Center tragedy had brought, they would all have acted just as swiftly as the FDA had to intervene. Unfortunately, a pharmacist tainted by corporate greed wasn't as easy to identify as a vial contaminated with mold, even though death came just as surely.

Pharmacists were dispensers of dangerous drugs, people were dying from dangerous drugs, pharmacists had rules to follow when dispensing these dangerous drugs, and social media was by now full of complaints about hurried working conditions within retail-chain pharmacies. This was all I knew, and I was going to grease the machinery of government agency a bit with these accusations.

A lawsuit is a petition brought before a judge, and it can be regarded in the same light as a "warning letter" from the FDA in that it's a letter of increased significance that might help motivate one to action. I didn't think the public had a year or two to wait until something was done to address the hurried pace in chain pharmacies, so I set about figuring out what type of lawsuit I needed to file. I was going to move forward with what would eventually become another "I told you so" moment.

My first legal hurdle was to prove that I had "standing," since a judge wouldn't hear or consider anything about the case unless I could prove that I had been injured either physically or financially by those I was accusing of wrongdoing. Without first proving standing, courts would be bogged down considering every simple dispute that came along when no actual harm was done. No lawyer will take your case if you cannot first convince them that you have been harmed, and by doing so, you will have achieved standing.

I was not being hurt by what was happening in retail-chain pharmacies; in fact, my own pharmacy was doing great. It seemed that the more chaotic retail pharmacy became, the busier I got. We were fielding all sorts of questions from strangers who had their prescriptions filled by chain pharmacies, and their need to know more brought new relationships to RC Compounding. We always told them to call their pharmacy and demand to speak with the pharmacist there. So, unsurprisingly, I spoke with several lawyers who all told me the same the same: "No harm here. You don't have standing."

So I looked to federal law to see if there was a way for me to continue with my claim. It turns out that if I could successfully argue that environmental law was being violated, I would be granted automatic standing. But could I prove that chain pharmacies were polluting the environment and endangering lives through the careless nature in which they were distributing poisons?

Since all drugs are poisons and, according to Paracelsus, "only the dose makes this not so," putting a label on a bottle full dangerous drugs and doing so without regard to dispensing laws seemed to me to be of greater risk to public health than if those drugs had been thrown directly into the Mahoning River and entered our water supply. After all, in this case, direct consumption is more dangerous than passive exposure. However, I'm not a lawyer, and I didn't want to gamble money on a federal case only to find that a judge didn't consider a drug to be a pollutant because it was swallowed instead of sipped. It made sense, though, for the brief period of time I contemplated it.

I had to look at state law and find a way to obtain standing. In Ohio, the Ohio Revised Code (ORC) is where most areas of our lives are regulated. It contains general directives that are passed along to state agencies who hammer out the specific rules that need to be followed. Our Board of Pharmacy is one such state agency, and their specific directives are contained in rules found in the Ohio Administrative Code (OAC). This is important because ORC and OAC have sections applicable to farming, industry, transportation, education, etc., not just pharmacy.

In my search, I found a law that would allow me to bring what is known as a "Public Action." I wouldn't have to prove that I'd been harmed but that all citizens in Ohio were being harmed because of the importance of the claim being brought. I could be the primary complainer, enjoining all Ohio citizens in the complaint if: 1) the claim involved an important issue, 2) the public cared about it, and 3) there was risk of further death should the court not decide in favor of the action being brought before them. Since I believed that our opioid addiction problem was one such important issue that people cared about, and deaths would continue if the courts failed to hear my argument, I felt that I had the standing I needed.

Once the court agrees that someone has been injured, they will consider the "relief" that the injured party is seeking. In essence, what is it that you want the courts to do? Since I had no specific prescription-dispensing incident to address and no specific patient who had been harmed, I had to claim that our Board of Pharmacy was not doing its job by not enforcing the rules. This was another hurdle for me because the law doesn't allow for an individual to direct the general activities of an agency, and without specific incidents of errors, I had an uphill battle.

Luckily, I found a way to petition a court to act regarding agency activity called a "Writ of Mandamus." The law allows a court to demand that an agency either do what the laws say it must do or stop doing what the law forbids. In my case, the law states that the Board of Pharmacy "shall act if it has reason to believe that laws are being violated," and I had a mountain of evidence, albeit not specific instances, to provide to the judges. Aside from chain pharmacies filling prescriptions day-in and day-out in under sixty seconds, which couldn't possibly comply with BOP rules, I had a petition, a pharmacists' resolution, newspaper reports, and social media rants by the thousands. Better yet, any judge could probably pull from their own experiences of having a prescription filled and say there was little compliance.

I now had a path forward and spent the next month or so writing the claim that named myself and the citizens of Ohio as petitioners against the agency that policed me: the Ohio Board of Pharmacy. I was, perhaps, about to set another record; I don't know whether a pharmacist had ever done something like this in Ohio. Who knows, maybe no pharmacist had ever done something like this before. On the other hand, there had never been circumstances like these before. Our opioid epidemic wasn't "normal circumstances," nor was a group of pharmacists suggesting that they're unable to dispense medications safely.

Many who I spoke with, family and colleagues alike, asked me to pause and think about what I was doing. As a pharmacist, suing a Board of Pharmacy, our policing agency, shouldn't be done lightly. I knew it was possible that my BOP could come after me with increased inspections, especially since my businesses were in their infancy and agency oversight was still being formulated. Plus, everyone seemed to be coming in to inspect us anyway. They would now have every reason to make life miserable for me. I crossed my fingers, hoping they saw some greater good in what I had been doing these past few years, remembered my visits prior to the New England Compounding Center tragedy, or would otherwise just see my action as one of the many that filled their daily plates. Either way, I prayed they wouldn't take offense at the offensive action I was about to bring. And I was about to bring it myself—"Pro Se" as they call it, Latin for "For Self"—since no lawyer seemed willing to help.

◆ ◆ ◆

20
CARLSON AND THE CITIZENS
OF OHIO VS. THE OHIO STATE
BOARD OF PHARMACY

I RESEARCHED AND WROTE THE COMPLAINT MYSELF. When I was ready, I dressed in a suit and tie and drove to the Mahoning County Clerk of Court's office in Youngstown, Ohio, to deliver the necessary copies of my lawsuit and pay a fee. The clerk asked if I was a lawyer, to which I answered, "No, but I did stay at a Holiday Inn last night." I was nervous and felt like I needed to break the ice with a joke.

I'm sharing my lawsuit now and in its entirety because of its absence elsewhere. Neither OPA nor APhA would publish it or mention it on social media. I expected as much at this point and took no offense. I was now siding with the public instead of trying to sway the profession, and Carlson now joined with all Ohio citizens. I no longer cared how pharmacists and their associations felt about my claim.

The greatest effort I had yet to put forth as a pharmacist—absent what this book extracts from me—was to sue my own professional policing agency. Later that night, when I was alone with my thoughts of what I may have just done to myself, my family, and possibly my profession, I teared up.

I print it here instead of summarizing and linking it to an addendum for all that this action means to me. Much of its content you
have already read, so feel free to breeze through it.

IN THE SEVENTH DISTRICT COURT OF APPEALS
STATE OF OHIO
MAHONING COUNTY, OHIO

STATE OF OHIO, EX REL	:
RAYMOND R. CARLSON, R.Ph.	: JANUARY—2018
	:
	:
	:
	:
Relator:	: Case No. _____
	:
vs.	: ORIGINAL ACTION IN
	MANDAMUS
	:
	: VERIFIED COMPLAINT
THE STATE OF OHIO BOARD	:
OF PHARMACY	:
77 South High Street, 17th Floor	:
Columbus, Ohio 43215	:
	:
Respondent	:

PETITION FOR PEREMPTORY
WRIT OF MANDAMUS

or

ALTERNATIVE WRIT OF MANDAMUS

INTRODUCTION

1. Relator, Raymond R. Carlson, R.Ph. (hereinafter referred to as "Carlson") brings this Petition for a Peremptory Writ of Mandamus or Alternative Writ of Mandamus in order to require that the Ohio Board of Pharmacy (hereinafter referred to as "The Board") immediately perform their lawful duties and demand that the Board enforce or cause to be enforced Section 4729 of the Ohio Revised Code, having been made aware that systemic violations of this chapter's provisions are occurring on a daily basis. Carlson has labored for several years within the profession, before the public, and most recently before the Board to warn of the impact and danger the public faces if the Ohio Revised Code and the Ohio Administrative Code Rules that pertain to the safe dispensing of prescription medication are not adhered to. In consideration of the opioid epidemic currently gripping Mahoning County and the State of Ohio, Carlson moves this Court for a Peremptory Writ of Mandamus or an Alternative Writ of Mandamus ordering the Board to examine evidence of violations of dispensing laws and to demand enforcement of the provisions of the Revised Code.

PARTIES

2. Relator Carlson is a resident of the State of Ohio, a 1985 graduate of Ohio Northern University Raabe College of pharmacy, is licensed and practices as a pharmacist in Mahoning County.

3. Carlson is the owner of RC Compounding Services, LLC located at 3030 Center Road, Poland, Ohio, 44514. RC Compounding is a pharmacy that dispenses compounded sterile and non-sterile drugs pursuant to patient-specific prescriptions. This business is licensed as a terminal distributor with the Ohio Board of Pharmacy and began operations in 2007.

4. Carlson is the owner of RC Outsourcing, LLC located at 102 East Water Street, Lowellville, Ohio, 44436. RC Outsourcing is an FDA Registered Outsourcing Facility and is licensed as a Wholesaler for Outsourcing Facility by the Ohio Board of Pharmacy. This business began operations in 2015 and provides only sterile dosage forms and without patient-specific prescriptions.

5. Carlson is a Past President of the Ohio Pharmacists Association (OPA) and Past President and Founder of the Eastern Ohio Pharmacists Association (EOPA). Carlson is a member of the American Pharmacists Association.

6. Carlson's work experience includes: large chain retail, small chain retail, independent, hospital, home infusion, consulting, and now self-employed in sterile and non-sterile compounding. Carlson is one of eight pharmacists in his family and his daughter is expected to graduate this May from ONU with honors.

7. Carlson brings this petition for a Peremptory Writ of Mandamus or Alternative Writ of Mandamus as a citizen and tax payer of Mahoning County and as that of a concerned pharmacist for the protection of pharmacy patients throughout the State of Ohio as well as for the lawful integrity of the profession.

8. The Ohio Board of Pharmacy (Respondent) has a principal place of business at 77 South High Street, 17th Floor, Columbus, Ohio 43215

9. Respondent is the single state agency in Ohio responsible for administering and enforcing laws governing the practice of pharmacy and the legal distribution of drugs.

10. The Board's mission requires that it "shall act efficiently, consistently, and impartially in the public interest to pursue optimal standards of practice through communication, education, legislation, licensing, and enforcement."

11. Section 4729.25 of the Revised Code requires that the Board "shall enforce, or cause to be enforced, this chapter. If it has information that any provision of this chapter has been violated, it shall investigate the matter, and take such action as it considers appropriate."

12. Section 3719.13 of the Revised Code states that "Prescriptions, orders, and records, required by Chapter 3719. of the Revised Code, and stocks of dangerous drugs and controlled substances, shall be open for inspection only to federal, state, county, and municipal officers, and employees of the state board of pharmacy whose duty it is to enforce the laws of this state or of the United States relating to controlled substances."

JURISDICTION

13. This Court possesses jurisdiction over the subject matter of this action according to Section 2731.02 of the Revised Code.

14. Based on this Petition and Verified Affidavit, there is no plain and adequate remedy in the ordinary courts of the law. Carlson petitions the state to "command the performance of an act which the law specially enjoins as duty" according to Section 2731.01 of the Revised Code.

15. Additionally, the State of Ohio's obligation to require the Board to perform its statutory duties is clear and it is apparent that no valid excuse can be given for not doing it and there is no plain and adequate remedy in the ordinary course of the law.

RELEVANT CODE AND REGULATIONS

16. The Omnibus Reconciliation Act of 1990 (H.R. 5835) (101st), also referred to as "OBRA-90," is a federal law passed by congress and a portion of that law is called "Drug Use Review." The law requires pharmacists to provide Patient Profiling of Information, Drug Utilization Review, and an Offer to Counsel before a prescription drug is dispensed to the patient in exchange for eligibility to receive federal funds.

17. The Board, subsequent to OBRA-90, expanded these services to all prescriptions filled and not just to those receiving federal funds in OAC 4729-5-18, et seq. The purpose of the "Drug Use Review" portion of OBRA-90 and the rules set forth in the Ohio Administrative Code are, amongst other things, to identify and reduce the frequency of patterns of fraud, abuse, and gross overuse of prescription drugs.

18. Carlson petitions this Court to require that the Board assess compliance with OAC Rules specifically promulgated in response

to the passage of OBRA-90. Both federal and state laws contain specific standards which would be difficult, if not impossible, for pharmacists to comply with given the number of daily prescriptions currently dispensed by pharmacists in retail and mail-order settings that seem rot with corporate metrics and insurance distractions.

19. Federal: As Passed By Congress and Signed Into Law on November 5, 1990

　　a. H.R. 5835 (101st): Omnibus Budget Reconciliation Act of 1990

　　　(g) DRUG USE REVIEW-

　　　(1) IN GENERAL-

　　　'(A) In order to meet the requirement of section 1903(i)(10)(B), a State shall provide, by not later than January 1, 1993, for a Drug Use Review Program described in paragraph (2) for covered outpatient drugs in order to assure that prescriptions (i) are appropriate, (ii) are medically necessary, and (iii) are not likely to result in adverse medical results. The program shall be designed to educate physicians and pharmacists to identify and reduce the frequency of patterns of fraud, abuse, gross overuse, or inappropriate or medically unnecessary care, among physicians, pharmacists, and patients, or associated with specific drugs or groups of drugs, as well as potential and actual severe adverse reactions to drugs including education on therapeutic appropriateness, overutilization and underutilization, appropriate use of generic products, therapeutic duplication, drug-disease contraindications, drug-drug interactions, incorrect drug dosage or duration of drug treatment, drug-allergy interactions, and clinical abuse/misuse.

20. State Rules Established By the Ohio Board of Pharmacy:

    a. The Ohio Administrative Code, as contained in OAC 4729-5-21, Manner of Processing a Prescription, requires the following:

        (A) A prescription, to be valid, must be issued for a legitimate medical purpose by an individual prescriber acting in the usual course of his/her professional practice. The responsibility for the proper prescribing is upon the prescriber, but a corresponding responsibility rests with the pharmacist who dispenses the prescription. An order purporting to be a prescription issued not in the usual course of bona fide treatment of a patient is not a prescription and the person knowingly dispensing such a purported prescription, as well as the person issuing it, shall be subject to the penalties of law.

        (B) A pharmacist when dispensing a prescription must:

            (1) Ensure that patient information is profiled pursuant to Rule 4729-5-18 of the Administrative Code;

            (2) Perform prospective drug utilization review pursuant to Rule 4729-5-20 of the Administrative Code;

            (3) Ensure that the drug is labeled pursuant to Rule 4729-5-16 of the Administrative Code;

            (4) Ensure that a patient is given an offer to counsel pursuant to Rule 4729-5-22 of the Administrative Code;

            (5) Ensure that a prescription is filed pursuant to Rule 4729-5-09 of the Administrative Code. (emphasis supplied)

    b. OAC 4729-5-18: Patient Profiles

    All pharmacies shall maintain a patient profile system which shall provide for immediate retrieval of information regarding those patients who have received prescriptions from that pharmacy.

(A) The dispensing pharmacist shall be responsible for ensuring that a reasonable effort has been made to obtain, document, and maintain at least the following records:

(1) The patient's data record, which should consist of, but is not limited to, the following information:

(a) Full name of the patient for whom the drug is intended;

(b) Residential address and telephone number of the patient;

(c) Patient's date of birth;

(d) Patient's gender;

(e) A list of current patient specific data consisting of at least the following:

(i) Known drug related allergies,

(ii) Previous drug reactions,

(iii) History of or active chronic conditions or disease states,

(iv) Other drugs and nutritional supplements, including nonprescription drugs used on a routine basis, or devices;

(f) The pharmacist's comments relevant to the individual patient's drug therapy, including any other necessary information unique to the specific patient or drug;

c. OAC 4729-5-20: Prospective Drug Utilization Review

(A) Prior to dispensing any prescription, a pharmacist shall review the patient profile for the purpose of identifying:

(1) Over-utilization or under-utilization;

(2) Therapeutic duplication;

(3) Drug-disease state contraindications;

(4) Drug-drug interactions;

(5) Incorrect drug dosage;

(6) Drug-allergy interactions;

(7) Abuse/misuse;

(8) Inappropriate duration of drug treatment; and

(9) Food-nutritional supplements-drug interactions.

(B) Upon identifying any issue listed in paragraph (A) of this Rule, a pharmacist, using professional judgment, shall take appropriate steps to avoid or resolve the potential problem. These steps may include requesting and reviewing an Ohio Automated RX Reporting System report or another state's report, pursuant to paragraph (D) of this Rule, and/or consulting with the prescriber and/or counseling the patient.

(G) A prescription, to be valid, must be issued for a legitimate medical purpose by an individual prescriber acting in the usual course of his/her professional practice. The responsibility for the proper prescribing is upon the prescriber, but a corresponding responsibility rests with the pharmacist who dispenses the prescription. Based upon information obtained during a prospective drug utilization review, a pharmacist shall use professional judgment when making a determination about the legitimacy of a prescription. A pharmacist is not required to dispense a prescription of doubtful, questionable, or suspicious origin.

d. OAC 4729-5-22: Patient Counseling

(A) A pharmacist or the pharmacist's designee shall personally offer to provide the service of counseling pursuant to paragraph (B) of this rule to the patient or caregiver whenever any prescription, new or refill, is dispensed. A pharmacist shall not be required to counsel a patient or caregiver when the patient or caregiver refuses the offer of counseling or does not respond to the written offer to counsel. If the patient or caregiver is not physically present, the offer to counsel shall be made by telephone or in writing on a separate document accompanying the prescription or incorporated as part of documentation, in a conspicuous manner that is included with the prescription. A written offer to counsel shall include the hours a pharmacist is available and a telephone number where a pharmacist may be reached. The telephone service must be available at no cost to the pharmacy's primary patient population.

(B) In the event a patient or caregiver accepts an offer to counsel or requests counseling, a pharmacist, or an intern under the personal supervision of a pharmacist, shall counsel the patient or caregiver.

Such counseling may include, but is not limited to, the following:

(1) The name and description of the drug;

(2) The dosage form, dose, strength, frequency, route of administration, and duration of drug therapy;

(3) The intended use of the drug and the expected action;

(4) Special directions and precautions for preparation, administration, and use by the patient;

(5) Common adverse effects or interactions and therapeutic contraindications that may occur, including possible methods to avoid them, and the action required if they occur;

(6) Techniques for self-monitoring drug therapy;

(7) Proper storage and disposal;

(8) Prescription refill information;

(9) Action to be taken in the event of a missed dose, and

(10) The pharmacist's comments relevant to the individual's drug therapy, including other necessary information unique to the specific patient or drug.

21. ORC 3719.05: Pharmacist May Dispense Controlled Substances—Prescriptions—Sale of Stock: "A pharmacist may dispense controlled substances to any person upon a prescription issued in accordance with section 3719.06 of the Revised Code. When dispensing controlled substances, a pharmacist shall act in accordance with Rules adopted by the State Board of Pharmacy."

FACTS

22. The May, 2011 edition of the Ohio State Board of Pharmacy News, which is "Published to Promote Compliance of Pharmacy and Drug Law," contains an article entitled *Corresponding Responsibility Is Needed More Than Ever*. The following excerpts add some clarity to the Board's expectations during a time when the seeds of our current opioid epidemic were being planted: "The pharmacist is often the last person who has the opportunity to make an independent judgment as to the legitimacy of the prescription and the patient. Both Ohio laws and rules and federal laws and regulations place a corresponding responsibility on the pharmacist to make that judgment and hold the pharmacist accountable for that judgment." As to the effort required and in consideration of distraction-free workplace conditions needed in order for a pharmacist to determine whether or not a prescription is written for a legitimate medical purpose, the article continues: "The fact that the pharmacist called the prescriber and was assured that the prescription was legitimate may not be enough. The pharmacist needs to look at the prescribing habits of the prescriber, the patient and his or her condition, and the dose of the drug or drugs being prescribed."

23. In 2013, Carlson received an insurance contract from a Prescription Benefit Manager ("PBM") at his pharmacy which had a clause stipulating that he was not allowed to "say anything negative" about the patient, physician, insurance company, or anyone associated with the care of the patient. Believing that this clause impedes a pharmacist's lawful duty to challenge the legitimacy of a prescription, and in response to a growing level

of frustration expressed to him by fellow colleagues, friends, and students, he founded the Eastern Ohio Pharmacists Association ("EOPA") which grew to 550 pharmacist members within one year. The annual membership meetings held at McMenamy's saw 200 pharmacists in attendance. EOPA represents pharmacists in Mahoning, Trumbull, Columbiana, Geauga, Lake, and Ashtabula counties. The theme of each meeting was opioid addiction and was covered by TV and print news.

24. Carlson has personally visited over 100 pharmacies in the six EOPA counties to speak with pharmacists and to encourage professional association as a means to address workplace conditions. Through conversation with pharmacists as well as internet surveys, the concerns of hundreds of pharmacists were revealed. EOPA used Survey Monkey to determine membership's most pressing issue to which members asked for management to recognize meal and rest breaks. A membership resolution requesting breaks was passed at their 2016 Annual Meeting.

25. At the March, 2017 annual Meeting of EOPA, members proactively debated a study being sponsored by the National Association of Chain Drug Stores (NACDS) in an attempt to prove that a pharmacy technician could check another pharmacy technician and dispense drugs in a manner equal to and in the absence of a pharmacist. EOPA overwhelmingly passed a resolution asking the Board to assess Rule compliance that pertain to lawful dispensing. Due to the reluctance of some EOPA officers to sign the association's letter to the Board, a citizen's petition requesting Board assessment of Rule compliance was circulated as an alternative and hundreds of signatures were obtained within several weeks.

26. Carlson emailed the Board to give notice that both the EOPA Resolution and Citizens' Petition were to be delivered personally to Board staff. Carlson hand delivered both in April of 2017 with accompanying information to support evidence that many pharmacists throughout the State of Ohio are frustrated and finding themselves unable to practice pharmacy as defined by law. The urgent nature of drug use issues, and in particular the opioid addiction epidemic that continues within Mahoning County and the State of Ohio, require immediate attention if even a portion of the problem is suspected to arise from violations of drug distribution laws, especially since such concerns have been brought to the attention of the Board. It is worth noting that there are no legal mandates for pharmacies in Ohio to report drug errors to the Board.

27. In conclusion, Carlson prays that this Court will consider the urgency of our County's and State's drug use problems and of the need to investigate through assessment all aspects of the distribution chain. Given the responsibilities that society has placed on the profession of pharmacy and of this petitioners efforts to bring to the attention of the Board of Pharmacy the concerns of many pharmacists that systemic violations of Drug Use Review Laws and Ohio Administrative Code Rules are occurring, the highly educated pharmacists from whom these drugs are dispensed in judgment of last resort must be considered to be worthy of the same assessments now being made of manufacturers, wholesalers, and physicians. Carlson brings this matter to the attention of this Court in good faith and with the belief that drug distribution laws are not being adhered to, that the Board of Pharmacy has been made aware of this through Professional Association

Resolution and Citizens' Petition, and that this matter is within the purview of this Court to intercede to ensure public safety as well as the integrity of a profession in whom, by law, the trust of the people is placed.

WHEREFORE, Relator requests relief from this Court as follows:

(A) The issuance of a Peremptory Writ of Mandamus or Alternative Writ of Mandamus requiring the Ohio Board of Pharmacy to enforce Section 4729.25 of the Ohio Revised Code; specifically, to investigate and assess compliance with dispensing laws as outlined in this petition within retail and mail order pharmacies; and

(B) If the Board determines that violations of federal or state law are occurring, to take any and all such actions that are appropriate to ensure the health and safety of individuals having prescriptions filled.

(C) The scheduling of a Hearing if found to be necessary,

(D) An award of court costs, other reasonable expenses incurred in maintaining this action, including reasonable attorney's fees.

Respectfully Submitted,
Raymond R. Carlson, R.Ph.

Exhibits A, B, C, D, and E are attached.

Soon after I filed my lawsuit, a local TV station contacted me for the scoop, and my filing appeared on the local news that evening. To this day, I believe it's the best visual summary of what this action was all about. It can be found at: https://youtu.be/Gy39oipikvE or by searching YouTube for "Ray Carlson TV 21 News Coverage."

In the middle of February 2018, I received a reply from then-Attorney General Mike DeWine's office in the form of a "motion to dismiss." The motion stated:

- I committed a procedural error in not serving them personally rather than by certified mail.
- I was advocating on behalf of a group of pharmacists and not the citizens of Ohio.
- I was trying to guide the activities of the Board in general.
- I was not considering actions already taken by the Board.
- I made no allegations involving specific instances of rule violations.
- Public-right standing exists "only where the alleged wrong affects the citizenry as a whole, involves issues of great importance and interest to the public at large, and the public injury by its refusal would be serious."

The motion closed with:

"While the relief requested by Carlson may be of interest to those involved in Carlson's professional advocacy group, the outcome of this case will not affect, and is not of great importance or interest to, the general public."

Signed, Yvonne Tertel
Assistant Attorney General

This is the part of the legal battle where the bickering occurs. My suit now entered a back-and-forth argument in the form of motions. All I was asking the Board of Pharmacy to do was go into chain and mail-order pharmacies and conduct an inspection to see whether lawful dispensing was taking place and if there was anything to substantiate the complaints coming from chain pharmacists about workplace conditions. Could these complaining pharmacists really fill one prescription a minute and do everything the law said they were supposed to do? Maybe the BOP would come out and say they'd found nothing. If that were the case, so be it; at least they would have looked.

Attorney General Mike DeWine, now Governor DeWine, didn't know that I didn't have the backing of my "professional advocacy group" and that I was merely passing on their complaint in the form of a resolution as evidence of the non-compliant situation pharmacists were finding themselves in. It was the only evidence of professional concern—an admittance of sorts—that I had at my disposal, and yet, ironically, it gave the impression that I was speaking directly on their behalf.

In my "opposition to their dismissal," I wrote:

"Carlson's Petition for a Writ of Mandamus asks for no new rules or mandates, nor does it ask for the Board to be inconvenienced by the performance of duties agreed to be discretionary. Instead, Carlson speaks on behalf of the public in the midst of an opioid scourge in order to require that the Respondent perform its statutory and administrative obligations. Carlson asks this court to reject OSBP's motion to dismiss on the grounds that the Ohio State Board of Pharmacy has the lawful duty to investigate, that these alleged rule violations are extraordinary and have a far-reaching impact on the public if allowed to continue."

In my reply, I also apologized for having not delivered the lawsuit personally instead of via certified mail. My biggest mistake, and one I wouldn't have made if I were a lawyer or had hired one, was that I didn't demand a hearing to state my case. At the time, I was confident and didn't feel I needed to. I wish I had taken the opportunity to speak and present a verbal explanation of what I was asking of the court; lawyer or not, I believe that the judges might have ruled differently. This was a tough call to make, so the regret doesn't hang too high over my head. Obtaining public standing was what threatened this case from moving forward.

I now had to wait for judges in the Seventh District Court of Appeals to decide the fate of my claim. I went back to work on the Liberty House in my free time and occasionally appeared on The *Louie B. Free Show* while I waited. Louie had become a dear friend and a source of encouragement and comfort. My brain cells needed a chance to decompress, especially since the few that were left wanted to think about the lawsuit and only the lawsuit. Everything else seemed trivial, and my efforts to hide this were taxing. So I kept to myself and let the months pass while I waited for the judges to decide my case.

Seven months after filing this action, I received my answer: "Petition is Dismissed."

The judges had the following to say:

"Relator [Carlson] is a licensed pharmacist who owns and operates his own pharmacy. He is also the founder of the Eastern Ohio Pharmacists Association (EOPA). The organization is comprised of pharmacists from Mahoning, Trumbull, Columbiana, Geauga, Lake, and Ashtabula counties. According to the Relator [the Board of Pharmacy], he founded the organization after he received an insurance contract from a Prescription Benefit Manager at his

pharmacy containing a clause which prohibited him to 'say any-
thing negative' about the patient, physician, insurance company,
or anyone associated with the care of the patient. He contends he
and other pharmacists view this clause as impeding the lawful
duty to challenge the legitimacy of a prescription. He also argues
workplace conditions in pharmacies are such that pharmacists
are unable to practice pharmacy in compliance with R.C. 4729-25
and its administrative regulations.

"Respondent is the single State agency in Ohio responsible
for administering and enforcing laws governing the practice of
pharmacy and the legal distribution of drugs. Its mission state-
ment is 'The State of Ohio Board of Pharmacy shall act efficiently,
consistently, and impartially in the public interest to pursue opti-
mal standards of practice through communication, education,
legislation, licensing, and enforcement.' Respondent must enforce
all laws relating to pharmacists and dangerous drugs and may
adopt rules and regulations as necessary to enforce the laws as
to the practice of pharmacy.

"While the opioid epidemic as portrayed by Relator is certainly
a very important issue, and the effects and harms related to it are
wide-reaching and encumbering, the alleged missteps made by
The State of Ohio Board of Pharmacy in the use of its discretion
do not rise to a level of a public harm that would be comparable
to Sheward. Therefore, Relator does not have standing to bring
the present suit."

I read the ruling with my heart in my throat, shed a tear, and then
read it again and again. "Oh no," I thought, "I should have gone with
environmental law for standing after all!"

The judge's opinion included the reasons why I was not given "public standing." This status had not been granted in fifteen years and was only awarded then for the constitutionally threatening nature of the claim being brought. The opioid epidemic didn't seem to rise to the high level of consideration the court thought necessary to grant a public standing claim. I disagreed and gave it my best shot, but failed.

What persisted across the Board's contention, their motion to dismiss, and the judge's ruling was that I had failed to "purport facts" by trying to articulate vague accusations without proof to support them. Our profession sensed the eight-hundred-pound gorilla in the room. We knew it was there, but no one would or could keep track of where it was sitting. The law clearly stated what pharmacists were expected to do before filling a prescription, the time needed to perform this didn't line up with the reality behind the counter, and people were dying as a result of what we had dispensed to them and the addictions we sold them. If only the cause was as clear as the consequences, public standing would have been granted if for no other reason than the numbers of dead.

I didn't have specific data to support my general claim of unlawful compliance, even though most in our profession knew in their heart of hearts that noncompliance was a problem. Pharmacists didn't have to report errors so there was nothing to collect and analyze. The Board of Pharmacy only responded if a citizen complained about a dispensing error. That would be public information. But how often does a patient call the BOP to report an error? They're usually given a bunch of coupons and an apology, the pharmacist is reprimanded, and the extent of the problem remains under the radar. We really didn't know how often and to what extent this was happening.

The judge continued:

"Even assuming Relator [Carlson] had standing, he could not sustain his claim. In the case of a petition for an emergency/ peremptory writ of mandamus, an appellate court's review of such a petition is narrowly prescribed by law. An appellate court can issue a peremptory writ of mandamus only 'if the pertinent facts are uncontroverted and it appears beyond doubt that [the relator] is entitled to the requested writ.'"

I understood the court's opinion, and I even agreed with it to a certain extent. Still, I felt the need to pay a lawyer $2,500 to tell me that I didn't have adequate grounds to appeal to our State Supreme Court.

That week, I went on the *Louie B. Free Show* and choked up on-air. I was an emotional wreck and in desperate need of the quiet time I always found necessary to help me cope.

In Asia, this is called "forest therapy," and it's often prescribed by physicians to treat anxiety. Simply shut everything off and sit in the quiet. Give your brain an opportunity to catch up with the chemicals it needs to make, and give yourself the opportunity to find a resolution to your current troubles before adding more.

◆ ◆ ◆

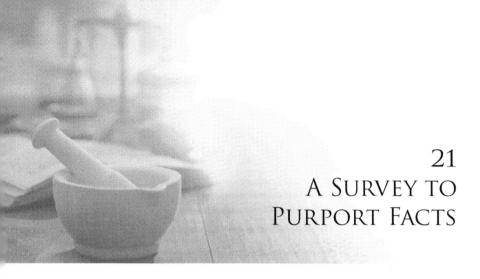

21
A SURVEY TO
PURPORT FACTS

THE SEVENTH DISTRICT COURT said that even if I had been granted standing, I failed to purport facts. Since I was fortunate enough to have a family member that could help me "purport," I called my sister-in-law, Toni Lynn Bisconti, Ph.D., who was a faculty member at the University of Akron's psychology department, and asked if it were possible for her to conduct a study for me. Soon after, Dr. Bisconti and I met at RC Outsourcing with two of her graduate students. She explained the rules behind such an undertaking and the risk of obtaining skewed results and an unsuccessful study if I involved myself in it.

Since my suit claimed that pharmacists were not following drug laws before handing drugs to citizens, I wanted to know if citizens agreed with that claim. If they were given a copy of the relevant law to read, would they then be able to state whether they felt that pharmacists were following the law in dispensing drugs?

It would ultimately take about nine months to complete the study. Shortly after the holidays, I received a text from my sister-in-law, Toni Lynn, informing me that the study was complete. "Merry belated-Christmas" she wrote, adding that the results would be emailed to me. I had built up a high tolerance for pharmacy-related anxiety and disappointment by this time but felt I had rejuvenated my spirit enough to allow me to accept whatever the results might be with grace.

The results of key parts of the survey are summarized here, and you can view the full survey in **Addendum 3:**

- 627 Ohio residents responded to the survey
- 67% have 1–3 prescriptions filled monthly
- 88% have prescription insurance and the remainder pay cash.
- 7% are filled at independent pharmacies, and 79.9% are filled at retail chain.
- 76% do not believe their pharmacist knows their name.
- 70% spend no time talking to a pharmacist, and 20% less than one minute.
- 75% either are rarely or never told about all categories of safe medication use.
- 41% are not clear as to what they are signing when they pick up their prescriptions.
- 75% do not believe an offer to be counseled on their drugs is bring made clearly to them.
- 61% were not aware that they were signing away their right to be counseled.
- 90% feel that pharmacists play an important role in thwarting drug abuse and misuse.

I was not surprised by the results because I had worked in a retail-chain pharmacy for many years, and I knew that what I was about to read would reflect what I had done and what I knew others were continuing to do in these environments. Life behind the pharmacy counter had only become worse since I last worked behind one, and I was shocked that the numbers were even worse than I expected. Would this survey have helped me in Carlson vs. Ohio BOP? Maybe not, but if the judges had considered each question as the Board of Pharmacy rule it represents, it would have been clear to them that rules were being violated. And in that case, Ohio laws says that the Board must investigate if it has knowledge of such violations occurring.

The judges might also have understood that all the suit was asking of them was to request that the Board investigate. There was no direct action requested other than to go in and take a look; if they saw what we suspected, how they tackled the problem would be up to them. But first, they had to recognize that there was a problem with the way chain pharmacists were filling prescriptions because of the amount of time their employers were giving them to do so. So many non-dispensing functions, called pharmacy metrics, were taking time away from pharmacists' ability to adhere to those functions that were meant to safeguard public safety.

Chain pharmacists are human, and there's only so much they can do in the time they are given. I wasn't able to abide by the law and the rules, either, and this is why I wasn't surprised by the survey's results. I can type and fill as fast as the best of them, but still, I'm only human, and the burdens are great and varied when dealing with the public and all the insurance problems this industry creates. On top of all that, toss in vaccinations, medication therapy management, constant computer training on new systems, an occasional hypochondriac, and the corporate desire for so many customers per day signing up for their app, and you have a pharmacist who is unable to fulfill what the laws tells them they have to do.

This survey addressed just the areas of dispensing that the public saw and experienced and did not include those that could only be found in the computers used to fill prescriptions. If we could dig into these areas, would we find the same level of compliance with the rule that states a pharmacist must enter pertinent notes into patient profiles? What about the practice standard that asks a pharmacist to call physicians and patients with concerns and then enter notes about these calls? What about how often warnings are simply overridden with a code? Although we couldn't obtain this type of information from patients themselves in this survey, a good IT person could find time stamps and determine how much time a chain pharmacist spends in thoughtful consideration of a pop-up warning before dismissing it.

Why would we think that chain pharmacists are given the time to dispense according to the rules if they aren't even given time to take a break? Instead, they eat on the run and work to find the bottom of the stack of baskets that the chain business models have forced in front of them.

This survey painted a picture of the chain workplace environment that we knew existed but, for one reason or another, failed recognize. One year after this survey was completed, our Board of Pharmacy would conduct a workplace survey of its own and end once and for all any misgivings for pharmacists, associations, and academia that a major problem exists, and our chain pharmacist colleagues need to be helped, not patronized. The eight-hundred-pound gorilla was now climbing around the room, and it could no longer be mistaken or overlooked.

With this survey in-hand, I teamed up with my friend Antonio Ciaccia, a senior advisor with the Ohio Pharmacists Association, to do a segment that would air on TV-5 WEWS News in Cleveland. Our conversation reached a large market, and, as Antonio and I would joke, he would hit them with a left punch and I with a right. The segment is titled "Pharmacy's Secret Crisis" and can be found at: https://youtu.be/5IkiWCXt7aA.

Throughout my journey through the minefield that is pharmacy, Antonio has been a constant source of support and guidance. As years pass and reflections sort out the details, the memory of our relationship will always be one of comfort, strength, and integrity. He says what he believes and works tirelessly to better pharmacy. I will always be grateful to him for the support and social media posts he gave me when it seemed no one else would.

Ideally, in a professional association, we're supposed to calmly and politely discuss the problems we face, propose solutions, vote on a solution, and then pass the chosen resolution to that problem onto the leaders to bring about change. This was not happening in the pharmacy world. Instead, chain pharmacists sat on the sidelines and allowed administrators to represent interests that were contrary to theirs. They allowed others to view the important role of dispensing dangerous drugs as though it were some old relic left over from previous generations that was without any clinical value. What they didn't understand was that retail dispensing is as clinical a practice as any, given the unique challenges it poses to those professionals who undertake it as the law says they should.

The addition of duties like vaccinations and Covid testing showed the fragility of pharmacy and the little time that pharmacists were being given to perform their duties, and the executive director of the Ohio Board of Pharmacy, Steven W. Schierholt, esq., was about to expose that fragility. The Ohio Board of Pharmacy conducted a workload survey in July of 2020 and released the results in April of 2021. This survey is the "purporting of fact" that came too late. Nevertheless, most everyone who cared about working conditions behind pharmacy counters were ecstatic that Steve had spearheaded this survey:

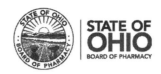

April 2021

Dear Ohio Pharmacists,

In July 2020, the State of Ohio Board of Pharmacy disseminated a workload survey to all pharmacists working in Ohio. The intent of the survey was to capture vital feedback on pharmacist working conditions in the state.

Capturing this data is important as pharmacist working conditions have been identified as a concern among licensees, state regulators (several of which have issued similar surveys i), and national organizations. For example, in 2019, the American Pharmacist Association conducted a national survey and reported "pharmacists' perceptions of their workload continues to increase in a number of settings." ii

The full results of Ohio's survey are included in this report, with freeform comments included separately (see Appendix I). The survey was sent out to 11,588 pharmacists and received 4,159 responses, a completion rate of 26.41%.

Moving forward, the data from this survey will be used to inform discussions regarding pharmacist practice in the state. The Board looks forward to working with a broad array of stakeholders to ensure Ohio's pharmacy professionals are working safely and in the best interest of the public's health.

Sincerely,

STEVEN W. SCHIERHOLT Executive Director

Of the 4,159 pharmacists who responded to the survey, 2,384 worked at a large chain or grocery chain pharmacy.

Question 1—I feel that I have adequate time to complete my job in a safe and effective manner.

726 Chain pharmacists Strongly Disagree

913 Chain pharmacists Disagree

265 Chain pharmacists were Neutral

(1,904 chain pharmacists out of 2,384 regarding patient safety behind their pharmacy counter)

Question 2—I feel that my employer provides a work environment that allows for safe patient care.

568 Chain pharmacists Strongly Disagree

872 Chain pharmacists Disagree

396 Chain pharmacists were Neutral

(1,836 chain pharmacists out of 2,384 regarding safe workplace conditions)

Question 3—I feel that my work environment has sufficient pharmacist staffing that allows for safe patient care.

758 Chain pharmacists Strongly Disagree

771 Chain pharmacists Disagree

384 Chain pharmacists were Neutral

(1,913 chain pharmacists out of 2,384 regarding not enough pharmacists)

Question 4—I feel that my work environment has sufficient pharmacy technician staffing that allows for safe patient care.

1,022 Chain pharmacists Strongly Disagree
    761 Chain pharmacists Disagree
    282 Chain pharmacists were Neutral

(2,065 chain pharmacists out of 2,384 regarding enough technician help)

These numbers continue with the same consistency for each of the questions the BOP asked. The ratios are similar, as are the conclusions one can draw from them.

The next few questions were:

Question 5—I feel that inadequate staffing at my pharmacy results in delays in patients receiving medications in a timely manner.

Question 6—I feel pressure by my employer or supervisor to meet standards or metrics that may interfere with safe patient care.

Question 7—I feel that the workload to staff ratio allows me to provide for patients in a safe and effective manner.

Question 8—I am given the opportunity to take lunch breaks or other breaks throughout the workday.

Question 9—I feel safe voicing any workload concerns to my employer.

One of the most telling questions was how many prescriptions a pharmacist was filling per hour.

1,571 answered that they fill prescriptions every 90 seconds of the day.
618 answered that they fill prescriptions every 60 seconds of the day.
235 answered that they fill prescriptions every 45 seconds of the day.
216 answered that they fill prescriptions every 30 seconds of the day.

The survey, complete with pie charts and bar graphs, can be found at https://www.pharmacy.ohio.gov/Documents/LawsRules/PWAC /CommitteeInformation/2020%20Pharmacist%20Workload%20 Survey.pdf or by Googling "Ohio Pharmacists 2020 Workload Survey."

The survey results also include specific pharmacists' comments. Reading through them, it's apparent that even after pharmacists escape from the chain pharmacy world, they still want to complain about it. So much of the passion and desperation in these comments come from a concern for public safety.

I have included just a few of the many pages of comments received by the Board:

I worked for a large chain until I simply could not accept the risk that they were putting on patients due to the focus on rx numbers and metrics at the cost of patient safety, not to mention the abuse of staff who are supposed to; It is totally unacceptable, unprofessional, and dangerous. I now refuse to work in that environment, but I based my answers on that experience. PLEASE do something to change this.

I worked for CVS for 10 years and my answers would have been the complete opposite. I constantly complained about staffing levels not being adequate for patient safety.

I worked in a large chain setting for 5 years post graduation. First as a floater, then staff, and finally a manager. I personally worked in ~50 pharmacies for this chain between PA and OH. There is absolutely no way I could have seen myself having a long career with this company. The working conditions were bad and only getting worse. There was a lack of pharmacist and technician hours, no lunch break, hard to go to the bathroom or eat, and verifying 400–500 prescriptions a day. In my opinion, it absolutely was not a safe environment and I worried constantly that we would make an error that would cause patient harm. The stress from the job was taking a toll on me physically and mentally. One year ago, I left that position and found an inpatient position with a smaller health system. Most days at my new position are much better with an outlier bad day. I don't know the solution to the community setting issues. I hope that this response is helpful in providing change for my colleagues.

I worked in a small chain; conditions were not horrible. When I gave Rx copies to RPhs at large chains, they would complain about the workload. The large chains seem to have the worst conditions. Its all about the money, money, money.

I worked in the retail chain environment for 35+ years. Its an awful environment. I am one of the lucky ones who escaped. I feel badly for all pharmacists and technicians still in that environment. All trust and credibility for me in that environment was lost. After I realized that no action was coming from corporate, state government, state pharmacy associations and the state board, I felt compelled to leave that environment. I was too loyal (and stupid) to think I could change the culture. Therefor, excuses were made up to get me out of the way of their agenda. Getting fired was a gift. There is truly no one on our side. In my current environment, I truly feel like an empowered pharmacist again, who can share valuable knowledge with patients, am able to really listen to them, and I am considered an important part of the community. I know many patients by name. I love them and they love me. That's the way it should be. I am treated as a professional. What a concept!

I worked in the retail setting for the first four years of my career. I have now been in the hospital setting for sixteen years. My answers to the above questions would have been dramatically different if I had taken this survey when I was a retail pharmacist. I am so glad the concerns of many of my colleagues may finally be addressed.

I worked retail before and there was not enough time to do all your work and not the staff to support the work. And definitely no lunch or other breaks.

I would be very interested in the Ohio BOP instituting a pharmacist to technician staffing ratio as other states have adopted. I feel it would force employers to adequately staff the pharmacy and help guarantee better support for the pharmacist without overloading them with work.

I would encourage the board to look into staffing seriously and have some regulatory enforcement based on the number of patients being cared for, acuity of care, and other factors that impact patient care. Corporates are clearly focusing on profits and numbers and not providing claimed "excellence" inpatient care (I.e. by not providing sufficient support staff to perform their job well); not only this will compromise patient safety; but, it will also impact negatively the outcomes of Pt therapy. If such issues are not addressed and reinforced by a regulatory body, pharmacy, and medicine in general, is becoming more of a business, than a healthcare institution established to provide patient care; defying the ethical commitment and oath we took, as healthcare professionals. Thank you

I'm blessed to work within a fantastic organization that values exceptional patient care over profit and volume metrics.

I'm concerned as flu season looms about administering immunizations during covid. We've started immunizing already but during flu season it obviously ramps up dramatically. We administer our immunizations in a small waiting room (about 7′ x 8′) and it's not uncommon to give 4 to 5 shots at a time to 5 different patients in there. I feel this is unsafe in the first place, but during covid, I'm more concerned. My employer has said we should start only allowing one person in the room at a time, but I feel policing the population of the waiting room during a busy day will be difficult. As is the case with most chains the priority on flu shots is high, due to the high margin. I'm glad we are immunizing so many people but giving 20 to 30 shots a day out of that small waiting room at the peak of flu season is kind of unsafe, especially when you account for our regular pharmacy traffic. I think if we want to keep making a bunch of money on flu shots, we should reinvest some of it in the facilities were immunizing in.

I'm glad this survey is being conducted. Pharmacists' work conditions are not acceptable, too many tasks, too many automatic prescriptions that were not requested by patients, hindering our ability to serve actual sick patients at the moment. Too many phone calls all while techs & pharmacists' hours are being cut. And the lack of breaks is another issue, working an average of 13 hours shifts, while not being able to take even a 15 min break. I hope this will result in real change. I love being a pharmacist; helping people with their meds; health. I try to accomplish this but the pressure to meet certain metrics makes it extremely challenging to just do our basic job!

I used to work for Rite Aid for 10 years and left because of the extreme lack of technician help—the extreme emphasis on giving patients immunizations whether or not they need them. Many pharmacists were giving each other unnecessary immunizations just to meet exceedingly ridiculous corporate goals. You were called out and ridiculed for not meeting goals. I thought is was actually dangerous for patient care—I expressed my opinion to management and felt I would be let go at some point.

These testimonials continue into perpetuity. This voluntary survey received eight or nine hundred comments, though it's impossible to tell what fraction of chain and mail-order pharmacists chose to add their own words. What should be concerning in all this is the number of chain pharmacists who outright fear for public safety, who are candid about the errors they commit, and who lay the blame directly at the feet of their employers. Based on this survey and the accompanying comments, there is clear and convincing evidence that the problem is the result of decades of indifferent administrators. And not just those who direct the business models of chain pharmacies, but also those who have passively allowed working conditions to deteriorate: legislators, Boards of Pharmacy, college deans and professors, professional association leaders, consultants, and the myriad of others whose job it is to see the big picture.

There are but a few chain pharmacies dominating retail pharmacy today, and they can be found in almost every city across the country that has a population of 5,000 residents or more. The smaller municipalities have all but lost their independent pharmacies and have become what is now referred to as "pharmacy deserts." In Ohio, there are about 250 cities with populations large enough to be blessed with access to a pharmacy, and the number of pharmacists in this survey alone, if spread out evenly, shows a state-wide patient-safety problem. Given that all chain pharmacies have similar, if not identical, business practices, our nation has a patient-safety problem. Media reports of dispensing errors, social media complaints about pharmacy experiences, and our nation-wide drug problem all point to a national problem.

These comments are a cry for help from pharmacists who mustered the courage to share their experiences, and while it would be difficult to determine the total number of pharmacists in Ohio who are working under these conditions, it would be safe to say that the problem is quite large. Even those who no longer work for chain pharmacies were eager to express near-hatred toward the chains that previously employed them. Their empathy for their colleagues who continue to labor under the conditions they felt fortunate to have escaped support the notion that the problem is one that individuals cannot fix themselves; they can only run from it. And yet, many took the opportunity to express their grievance in this survey.

These comments contain admissions that go beyond our general concerns of simple dispensing errors: errors that involve either the wrong patent, wrong drug, or wrong directions. These are the assembly-line type of errors that happen because of haste, and since chain pharmacists are admitting that these types of errors are likely, they're essentially admitting that they work on an assembly line and that all the duties attached to proper dispensing have been removed to complete only the most nominal of tasks.

In these comments, chain pharmacists didn't express concern about not being able to gather the twelve pieces of patient information the law requires before filling a prescription or not being able to go over the twenty-one pieces of drug information the law encourages them to provide. Instead, they fear making the simplest of errors, such as putting the right pills in the wrong bottle. When chain-pharmacy business models have burdened pharmacists to such an extent that even these most basic of dispensing tasks are threatened, how can they have the time to comply with other mandates that are more time-consuming? Without chain corporations giving their pharmacists the time to ensure basic safety, how can they claim their business models comply with the law?

This brings us to the conversations that go beyond the obvious danger of being given the wrong pill or handed someone else's prescription. Sure, it's easy to spot an error when a patient returns home, opens their pill bottle, and notices that their medication is a different shape or color, but will they understand the danger when chain pharmacists don't take the time to look at a patient's other prescriptions? A drug, even if dispensed "correctly," can still cause harm if a patient has previously been prescribed a medication that's not safe to take with another.

The *Chicago Tribune* conducted an investigative study in 2016 by purposefully presenting two prescriptions to pharmacies in the Chicago area that should never be taken together:

> *"In the largest and most comprehensive study of its kind, the Tribune tested 255 pharmacies to see how often stores would dispense dangerous drug pairs without warning patients. Fifty-two percent of the pharmacies sold the medications without mentioning the potential interaction, striking evidence of an industrywide failure that places millions of consumers at risk.*
>
> *"CVS, the nation's largest pharmacy retailer by store count, had the highest failure rate of any chain in the Tribune tests, dispensing the medications with no warning 63 percent of the time. Walgreens, one of CVS' main competitors, had the lowest failure rate at 30 percent—but that's still missing nearly 1 in 3 interactions.*
>
> *"In response to the Tribune tests, CVS, Walgreens and Wal-Mart each vowed to take significant steps to improve patient safety at its stores nationwide. Combined, the actions affect 22,000 drugstores and involve additional training for 123,000 pharmacists and technicians.*
>
> *"'There is a very high sense of urgency to pursue this issue and get to the root cause,' said Tom Davis, CVS' vice president of pharmacy professional services."*

Drug-drug interactions are but one area of patient safety that proper compliance with dispensing rules would ensure. What about patients who have a condition that would exclude the use of one drug from being used to treat another condition? And what about those patients who have medical devices, allergies, prior reactions to drugs, or are taking over-the-counter medications that are contraindicated with taking a new drug? These considerations and many more are why pharmacists need to obtain full, correct patient information when a prescription is presented.

Evidence was mounting that chain pharmacies and the independent pharmacies that were forced to follow their business models were failing to follow dispensing laws, yet our profession still denied that this was the case. Academia continued to bash retail dispensing and push its clinical agenda of hospital- and Medication Therapy Management (MTM)-focused roles, professional associations declined to publish articles or even repost these media reports on social media, and agencies found themselves too bogged down with other problems to afford the manpower necessary to contain such widespread and seemingly accepted workplace conditions. No pharmacy-related entity, with all their elected, sworn-in, and educated thinkers, pushed for our government representatives to consider that dispensing laws were being broken.

Administrators, agencies, academia, and associations will not admit that patients are being harmed unless there are enough basic errors like "wrong drug" and "wrong patient," even though more complex issues like missed personal interactions, missed addictions, and adverse drug reactions are just as important as missed patient names. To make matters worse, even the simplest of errors doesn't have to be reported to the Board of Pharmacy and made public. The lack of evidence is a self-fulfilling prophesy: officials won't go out on a limb to correct patient-safety issues due to the lack of damning evidence of patient-safety issues. Meanwhile, the public endures addiction, disease, and adverse reactions because these types of errors aren't obvious enough to draw the attention of those who could have ended them.

If a patient is injured, they can question how good a chain pharmacy has been at obtaining the patient information they're supposed to. They can ask how many prescriptions a pharmacy is filling per hour to ascertain how much time is spent considering the appropriateness of the drugs they're dispensing. They can subpoena to see counseling logbooks to know whether that pharmacy has the time to talk to patients. They can ask to see if warnings were overridden when their prescription was filled and request a printout of their profile to see if the pharmacist had taken the time to enter any notes specific to that or any other dispensing activity. Being educated about the law means the public has recourse when the law isn't being followed. No jury is necessary when the injured party makes a claim in a letter to the offender and that letter is written in such a way as to remove the information asymmetry that was required for the offense to be perpetrated to begin with.

The comments in this survey come directly from chain pharmacists themselves and provide a place for an injured individual to start asking questions. Pharmacists simply cannot ensure public safety when their working conditions are so dire, and patients can bring action that ferrets out the deceit if they educate themselves about drug-drug interactions, drug-disease interactions, and polypharmacy to see the multitude of dangers that a company had carelessly exposed them to. If Googling individual drug information is too difficult or complex, ask someone more learned to run a scan of all medications. Such efforts will reveal a variety of warnings categorized as mild, moderate, or severe, as well as what one might experience if the drugs were taken together.

With knowledge, a patient can determine if the drugs they have been prescribed have caused the harm described in the literature.

Include this drug information in a letter to the chain or mail-order pharmacy responsible for filling the prescription, include a notice to subpoena other information that would support a claim of general failure to comply with dispensing laws, and see what they do. The people have the power to make change if they know what to ask for.

The comments on this survey admitting the reality of pharmacy conditions and the threat it represents to public safety are of greater value than any evidence I might present. If you're interested, I encourage you to visit the Ohio Board of Pharmacy website to read the full comments for yourself. The Board asked for "any additional comments a pharmacist would have thought to be helpful," and they received more than they expected.

Years of silence from chain pharmacists finally came to an end when they found the courage to respond to an anonymous solicitation of their opinions. I likened their testimonials to the TV interviews chain pharmacists would do while wanting their faces blurred and voices garbled. Still, they had the courage to admit that patient lives were in danger, and I applaud them.

The change that is now needed to protect the safety of citizens might now come too late to be done at the hands of chain pharmacists themselves. Instead, suffering has reached the level that now calls on the public to take action. Now it is up to the public to demand change through the courts. The U.S. death rate can no longer wait for committees to meet and boards to convene, and we certainly cannot trust that corporate pharmacy will act. No chain pharmacy, association, agency, or college will admit now that the root of the problem has been the lack of adherence to OBRA-90 laws. By doing so, they would be admitting that they said nothing about the rule violations at a time when the suffering could have been prevented. Now that the cat is out of the bag, and damage has been done and continues to be done, resolution now lies in the public hands. And just as the fate of compounding pharmacy was in question for the moral hazards it committed, so too is retail pharmacy for what it has done or what it has failed to say to prevent it.

◆ ◆ ◆

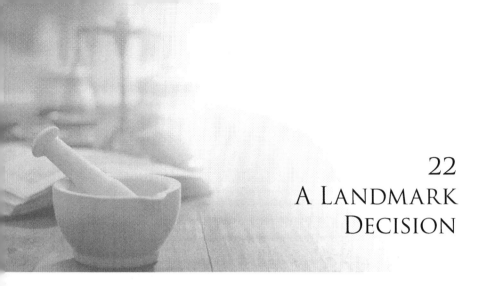

22
A LANDMARK
DECISION

My EFFORTS TO BRING RETAIL-CHAIN-PHARMACY workplace
conditions to light were frustratingly ahead of the curve by several years, and now, in 2021, I was beginning to experience some
vindication. Citizens residing in the two counties to the north of
me, who would not only have "standing" on this issue, but also
the money to hire the lawyers, filed a lawsuit against five major
chain pharmacies, and the claim was basically the same as I was
making to our board of pharmacy. They were asking for damages
that occurred because of violations that I was asking our board to
stop. The issue had not changed. The public threat I'd attempted to
bring to light was still present. But now, it would be the public that
would make the same argument in a court of law and before a judge
who was much more familiar with our nation's opioid epidemic,
Judge Dan Polster.

I learned about this new legal effort when I received a call from an
attorney with the law firm that was representing Lake and Trumbull
Counties here in Ohio. They had filed a lawsuit against five major chain
pharmacies, and they wanted to get my take on the issues affecting

chain pharmacists. Over the course of several hours, I gave the best explanation I could of OBRA-90, Ohio law, and what I believed was going on behind chain pharmacy counters. When the session ended, with my mouth dry and head pounding, I went back to work with a resurgence of energy.

The lawsuit was Trumbull and Lake Counties vs. CVS, Walgreens, Walmart, Rite Aid, and Giant Eagle—in a "public nuisance claim," of all things. Other municipalities watched it closely, since a suit like this had never been brought before. No matter the outcome, though, some measure of vindication was mine, since my suit against our Board of Pharmacy made the same basic contention this suit was now making. The suit claimed that these five chain pharmacies created a "public nuisance" in the way they controlled the distribution of prescription pain pills and that the reckless way they did it contributed to the opioid epidemic. Rite Aid and Giant Eagle settled out of court without admitting wrongdoing. The others would battle it out. The trial was set for October 2021, and after many delays, it appeared as though it was going forward.

It's probably a coincidence that these two counties are in our EOPA district, but be that as it may, it was nice to know that chain dispensing problems had first been pointed out in northeastern Ohio several years earlier. It seemed only fair that this bellwether case was happening here and that sweet justice might finally arrive after years of struggle.

No one had yet sued a chain pharmacy for its role in the opioid epidemic, and this must have made every corner of the pharmacy profession shudder with anticipation. Of course, you'd never have known it, given the lack of chatter on social media and professional association websites. I'm not sure why pharmacy kept silent as the case moved forward since it was corporate chain pharmacy on trial and not individual chain pharmacists. Part of me expected that everyone in pharmacy would be cheering. So why didn't they?

Two counties in Ohio had the courage to contend that it was chain business models that were responsible for the chaos behind the pharmacy counter and that individual pharmacists were only pawns in their game, as we had suggested they were. Finally, corporate pharmacy was being called out for the moral hazards their CEOs, supervisors, marketing staff, and business developers had engaged in. The failures of state pharmacy associations and our national APhA to mention and support the changes that could come from this suit meant that they had lost yet another opportunity to open their association doors to potential chain pharmacist members.

It no longer mattered to me what other pharmacists thought of the allegations I'd been making, what any professional association thought of the embarrassing light I was shedding, or the lack of importance that academia placed on "simple dispensing." All that mattered to me was that the people were now going to have a chance to hear and understand the law and listen to witnesses tell their stories. A jury of our peers would determine if the conduct alleged was lawful or not. It was a $650 million decision on the line for the losers.

Oh, to have been a fly on the wall in the courtroom! Or, even better, to have been able to call a CEO to the witness stand! I had my own line of questioning down pat at this point, and I wouldn't have allowed them to escape without giving the jury a clear understanding of what they had perpetrated. Among the questions in my arsenal:

* Did you allow your pharmacists time with the computer and the patient, assist with adequate technician staffing in order for them to use their six-to-eight years of education before deciding whether it was okay to fill a prescription?

- Did you allow your pharmacist the time to make eye contact with a patient, have a conversation, and mention some of the warnings that either they or a technician had overridden with a passcode?
- Did you or did you not pressure your pharmacists with a screen that changed colors when "time was up"?
- Did you required your pharmacists to achieve flu-shot quotas that would have caused them to ask more about vaccinations than about drug interactions and side effects?
- Did your pharmacists have enough time to pick up on the fact that OxyContin was showing addictive properties? Were there no notes of concern about OxyContin in the profiles of the patients to whom you dispensed this drug?
- Please give the jury a possible business-model scenario, any scenario at all, that would allow the seventy-five steps of proper dispensing to be done in under sixty seconds.
- Please describe for the jury your take on the meaning of "equal and corresponding responsibility" and what constitutes a drug being used for a "legitimate medical purpose."

There isn't a single licensed chain pharmacist in the state that I would call to the stand to testify—only their bosses, district supervisors, board members, and CEOs. The pharmacies, not the pharmacists, were to blame here.

Yes, chain pharmacists should have organized in some way to speak out or at least comfort their fellow colleagues, but remember, they had no organizations of their own. They would have had to first tear down the barriers within larger pharmacy organizations and compete with other, well-entrenched interests. It must have seemed like an overwhelming task to push aside the articulate clinical interests of hospital pharmacists, academia, or chain members whose dues were paid by their employers. Without a national organization of their own, conditions crept toward despair until no amount of pain and suffering could move them. It only made their distaste for professional association life that much more bitter.

You can call the individual pharmacist culpable to a certain extent, but it was corporate pharmacy on trial now. And on November 23, 2021, it was corporate pharmacy that would be found guilty of creating a public nuisance, as the Associated Press reported:

CVS, WALGREENS AND WALMART RESPONSIBLE FOR ROLE IN OPIOID CRISIS, OHIO JURY SAYS

JOHN SEEWER
Associated Press

CLEVELAND—CVS, Walgreens and Walmart pharmacies recklessly distributed massive amounts of pain pills in two Ohio counties, a federal jury said Tuesday in a verdict that could set the tone for U.S. city and county governments that want to hold pharmacies accountable for their roles in the opioid crisis.

Lake and Trumbull counties blamed the three chain pharmacies for not stopping the flood of pills that caused hundreds of overdose deaths and cost each of the two counties about $1 billion, their attorney said.

How much the pharmacies must pay in damages will be decided in the spring by a federal judge.

It was the first time pharmacy companies had completed a trial to defend themselves in a drug crisis that has killed a half-million Americans over the past two decades.

The counties were able to convince the jury that the pharmacies played an outsized role in creating a public nuisance in the way they dispensed pain medication into their communities.

"The law requires pharmacies to be diligent in dealing drugs. This case should be a wake-up call that failure will not be accepted," said Mark Lanier, an attorney for the counties.

"The jury sounded a bell that should be heard through all pharmacies in America," Lanier said.

During the trial, corporate chain pharmacies argued that it wasn't just chain pharmacies that were filling vast quantities of prescriptions for addicting drugs; independent pharmacies filled their fair share, if not more. While this might be true to some extent, the "bread-and-butter" maintenance prescriptions that independent pharmacies had once filled for their customers were taken away by chain pharmacies which signed contracts with insurance companies (PBMs) stating that they could fill prescriptions and perform all dispensing duties for one dollar's worth of reimbursement. By doing so, they left independents to dispense classes of drugs like painkillers and antibiotics that might not otherwise have represented normal pharmacy dispensing patterns.

With the gravy prescriptions gone and handed over to hurried chain pharmacists and mail-order facilities, there was little left to make a living on. Independent pharmacies didn't own cost-saving mail-order pharmacies like the chain pharmacies did, so there was no way they could compete with a contract calling for adherence to all laws for one dollar while still paying their overhead. A chain pharmacy could make up those loses at their mail-order facilities. Or, worse yet, if they *owned* the insurance company, they made big money through the "rebates" (kickbacks) they received from drug manufacturers if they allowed their drug into their formularies.

The funny money received on one end propped up losses on another. These financial games created the chain-pharmacy business model that independents had to adjust to if they wanted to keep the lights on and continue to feed their families. Did independents venture into moral hazards in the way they dispensed opioids to the public? Most certainly! If they were lucky enough to be one of the last remaining mom-and-pop stores to survive, they would also need to fill a prescription every sixty seconds in defiance of dispensing laws just to compete. You get what you pay for, and chains were determining the pay.

This court decision sparked joy in me for my profession, and yet, there was almost no talk about it on social media. I saw very few posts with no likes and no shares, just as I saw when my lawsuit became public. There was no conversation about the merits of either even though both were attempting to bring a public good, and no matter the profession or industry, public safety trumps everything always.

I understood why few in the pharmacy world would want to say anything about our profession being considered a public nuisance, but this was a victory for us. For years, I had maintained that the public would eventually fix what we failed to, and now, they had made a $650 million step toward that. If pharmacists couldn't speak out about the eroding compliance within dispensing laws, the people eventually would when they'd had enough of it. Only now, pharmacists and pharmacies wouldn't be the captain of the ship. Just as with the New England Compounding Center tragedy, the badges would step in, and at that point, you've lost control of your destiny.

◆ ◆ ◆

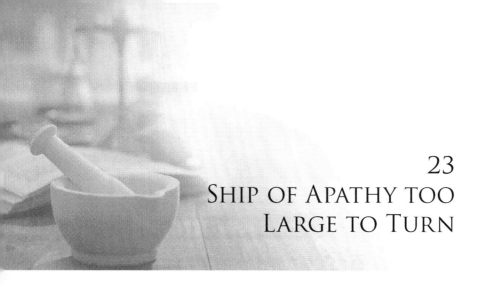

23
SHIP OF APATHY TOO
LARGE TO TURN

IN MY TWENTY-FIVE-YEAR WAR to bring to light the problems behind chain pharmacy prescription counters and the corporations responsible for creating them, I learned that there were far too many players involved to think the problem would easily resolve itself. I spoke with many lawyers, pharmacists, news reporters, radio hosts, legislators, addicted citizens, educators, and counselors, and each time I thought I had made progress, there was no returned call, no interview, no coverage. I can handle outright rejection, but what frustrated me most was not doing a podcast after an initial conversation, reading a story riddled with errors because the reporter was hurried, or seeing the lack of "likes" on a post. If Zig Ziglar's claim that "we are where we are because that is exactly where we want to be" is true, our ship is heading in the direction it is because many seem to be steering it in that direction.

I was glad that Lake and Trumbull Counties won their lawsuit and were about to receive $650 million. I was also kicking myself for not having hired a lawyer myself several years earlier during my own lawsuit. A couple of years before I filed my suit against the Ohio

Board of Pharmacy, I brought my concerns to our Mahoning County prosecutor's office. I thought I had stumbled upon something related to our opioid problem here at home, and I wanted to run the idea past them to see if the county might want to try to get back some of the prescription monies they had been spending on employees over the years.

Their office is located on the fifth floor of our county courthouse in downtown Youngstown, and apparently, it's a floor no one is supposed get off at. I did not know this and there were no signs posted. So I made my way to the fifth floor and was met by an attorney as I exited the elevator, and he asked if he could help me. I said, "I just want a couple minutes to talk to a prosecutor about something I believe is important."

"Did you make an appointment?" he asked.

"Well, *no* . . . I just wanted to see what someone thought about this," I replied. It was obvious that no one wanted to talk to me, and I was verbally pushed back into the elevator. With a spark of inspiration, I turned around and said, "My brother-in-law is Judge Durkin who runs the Mahoning County Drug Court, and he told me to stop by with this information."

The next thing I knew, I was sitting at a table with an uninterested lawyer, showing him the 150 pages of laws, chain pharmacist complaints, and other similar suits, that I'd brought along to make my point. I could tell he was going to toss everything in the trash shortly after I left. He didn't realize it then, but he'd just tossed $650 million away. Now mind you, I had never sued anyone before, and suing my BOP was an idea still a couple years away. But I was given the impression by this attorney that I was a troublemaker of some sort. And it was the same impression I had received months prior when I called our county's human resource department to ask for a copy of our county's prescription drug benefit contract with a PBM. I was made to feel like I was someone who was up to no good . . . and good was the only thing on my mind.

A couple of years after this run-in with the prosecutor's office, I was appointed to serve as foreman of our county's grand jury. Every Thursday for three months, I got on and off the elevator at the fifth floor, walked past prosecutors' offices, and signed paperwork for the indictments we heard during the day. Most of the cases involved drug offenses, and the fifth floor's busy pace was due to prosecuting them. In the back of my mind, I kept thinking of the statistic that pharmacies were responsible for 75 percent of addictions; at the time, I was writing my own suit against our Board of Pharmacy. I empathized with those who had done wrong just as much as those bringing them to justice. But where was justice to be found for those who became addicted due to careless dispensing practices? I had attempted to deliver the head of the snake to our county prosecutors two years earlier, and the effort was dismissed.

On the same lines, and at the same time I had first offered concerns to the county prosecutor's office, I stopped at the Mahoning County Commissioners' office just a few floors down on my way out. I had a packet for them as well. I talked to the secretary for a while and asked her to give this information to one of our county commissioners and to please call me to arrange a meeting. They never called. Months later, I sat at a table and ate dinner with a county commissioner at a fundraiser for Senator Schiavoni, who was running for governor at the time, and I explained once again what I had dropped off at her office. I told the commissioner that I never received a call and sensed that they thought I was a troublemaker looking to sue them. The idea of a well-meaning citizen showing up out of the blue to speak with them about doing good was apparently too incredible to take seriously. I would have similar conversations with BOP members, the president of the each of the major pharmacy associations: NCPA, OPA, and APhA, as well as with legislators, radio talk-show hosts, and my mailman. Change was not mine to instigate.

How does someone get past the appearance of ulterior motives to jump into the problem-solving portion of the process? Who cares how the fire began; it needs to be extinguished, and it can be no one's fault if it's everyone's fault. There is always time to go back and point fingers, but first, stop the bleeding. If we all turned our backs on the law, so be it, but it was now the time to turn around and fix things.

When looking at the size of the ship and the many parties involved in setting its course, remember the portion of OBRA-90 laws that require each state to establish a Drug Use Review Board. The first portion of the law mandates what a pharmacist is supposed to do when filling a prescription; the second establishes a review board to monitor how those activities are impacting the community. A group of physicians and pharmacists are required to look at prescription data received by the state and determine if there are patterns of abuse or misuse. They're also required to file an annual report recapping year-to-year trends. All states that receive federal money for prescriptions need to have these anti-abuse features in place, and they were given three years to do it. So, why were opioid trends not picked up and reported in the fifteen years that these professionals had to look at the data?

The Ohio Department of Medicaid website includes the meeting minutes from the state's review board, which meets quarterly. Each meeting averaged about an hour—many, for even less—and there was no mention of concern about increased use of opioids, no upward trends to act on, just jibber-jabber over coffee and exchanging pleasantries during that decade when timing mattered most.

Other states missed it, too. They were looking at data, and lots of it, but who in their right mind would question the "legitimacy" of the prescriptions that constituted the data? The members of these committees all assumed that all laws and rules pertaining to dispensing were being followed and that the data they were looking at had already passed society's lawful litmus test. They assumed wrong; they never questioned the legitimacy of the data by first questioning the legitimacy of the prescriptions.

One would think that a "Drug Use Review Board" not sounding any alarms as millions became addicted would be front-page news, but it wasn't. Why? Because certain individuals on these boards would be shamed? Names we don't know or care about. The past and present members of these boards learned about the epidemic at the same time everyone else did. The system needs to be fixed, yet no one is willing to step in and say so. Looking at the system and not the individuals would have been one more way to shine light on the fact that legal dispensing laws were not being followed. If they had been, the misuse and abuse that caught everyone by surprise would have been caught.

It's important for people to understand how legitimate pain patients were being hurt. Pharmacists had to contend with an employer-sponsored volume that prevented them from stopping illegitimate and unnecessary prescriptions, and so, they were mixed in with the legitimate and necessary prescriptions. As far as anyone was concerned, everything seemed legit. Patients could walk out of chain-pharmacy doors without talking to anyone. The chains created the anonymity that turned people into data. Now that chain pharmacy had been declared a public nuisance in two Ohio counties, I'm certain our Board of Pharmacy sat up in their chairs remembering the petition I'd brought to them four years earlier.

There is no other way to characterize the behavior of those who gave us this title other than to say that it had become the "new normal" and because of this it was able to escape detection for so long. Colleges and professional associations had been downplaying the importance of "drug dispensing" for years, characterizing it as an activity that is beneath us—one that simply involves counting by fives. Is it possible that their characterizations stemmed from the fact that they had no idea of the sheer size of the laws/rules that applied to dispensing or understood the responsibilities our BOP had in enforcing them? Had they never read the laws from the perspective of the people well enough to appreciate the dangers these very laws warned us of?

We were repeatedly told that "dispensing is dead." This notion was being pounded into the heads of college students. "Pharmacists belong in an office or cubical delivering clinical information," we heard all the time. Did they mean the same information patients could obtain through Google? What about our ability to see a patient's big picture because of repeated visits by walking, talking humans or our ability to articulate the importance of proper drug consumption, repeatedly, in a funny way, in a charming way, in a humane way? What about making eye contact with someone who was visiting five different doctors to obtain a controlled substance? What about gathering information on the front end, taking the time to consider a patient's profile before bottling a drug, and talking to the patient directly through drug counseling?

Instead of recognizing the plight of chain pharmacists and acting in ways that could help them, professional associations and academia pushed for ridiculous laws that only made their situation worse. One such law required pharmacists to perform Medication Therapy Management (MTM), which meant that when a person was taking several medications incorrectly, a pharmacist could make money by billing a patient's insurance for services that the pharmacist should have rendered at the time the prescription was originally filled.

An entire industry of MTM companies sprang up, making money on the seminars that trained pharmacists on how to use the new computer software needed to bill for this service. At one point, I heard that pharmacists were paid twenty-five dollars even if the patient phone call went unanswered. One can imagine all the moral hazards that came into play with something that should never have been needed to begin with. MTM is nothing more than the Drug Utilization Review that OBRA-90 calls for, and the fact that insurance companies pay only one dollar to fill a prescription shouldn't mean that this portion of dispensing law should be skipped, especially when an addictive drug is involved.

They started teaching MTM in colleges instead of returning to the laws the people (lawmakers) had already passed and expected us to follow. So what if a chain pharmacy had diminished the value of dispensing to the dollar it would accept from an insurance company for filling the prescription. Did academia assume that the chains had made up the losses elsewhere in their business models and kept the dispensing service propped up to maintain lawfulness? Or might they have thought the laws had been tossed in the trash because compliance with it generated only one dollar of income. I feel for all the educators who heard the stories coming from students returning from summer intern jobs at chain pharmacies without considering that there might be unlawful, if not unmoral, conduct taking place, and just as chain pharmacists themselves were unable to do, they continued to teach as others had told them to.

The laws of proper dispensing are too lengthy and complex for our colleges and associations to discount its importance to the people. By dismissing the key elements of dispensing practices in the real world of retail pharmacy, academia does a grave disservice to students by denying them the opportunity to practice in a way that the law states is as clinical as any they would experience in a cubicle or beside a hospital bed. The grandeur they expect when they finally become licensed pharmacists is replaced with disappointment and despair. What a shock it must be for our new graduates to leave the comforts of a college that sold them on clinical tasks, only to enter the unsafe conditions expressed in all the comments of our BOP's survey.

Here is the "greater good" behind professional associations and why not participating in these associations contributed to our opioid epidemic. Say a pharmacist spots something, maybe a sign of addiction or maybe a beneficial side effect like what we discovered with Avastin, and that pharmacist happens to mention this to another pharmacist who was about to mention the very same observation. The next thing you know, a group of pharmacists is admitting to the same revelation. It gets discussed, people vote, and someone prepares a resolution and hand-delivers it to their state association for consideration. Lo and behold, pharmacists from around the state are noticing the same thing. . . . And up the food chain it goes to APhA to see if it's just something in Ohio's water or if other states are seeing similar trends. If so, that issue is passed on to legislators—and change happens. It's lawful democracy, it's redress, and it's what is expected from an individual who has spent $250,000 and six-to-eight years on an education.

Not only did our failure to make use of democracy prevent us from catching the addictive properties of OxyContin, but also, a higher-strength version entered the market while we failed to act. A profession that is bound to a law like the one passed in 1990 to spot drug abuse and misuse is no profession at all if corporate pharmacy creates a public nuisance and takes away the professional's ability to detect such dangers. The public nuisance must be removed, and the professionals must be allowed to return to doing what the people expect from them. Anyone who reads and understands OBRA-90's Drug Use Review can see that if it had been followed as written, the opioid epidemic could have been prevented. The fact that it wasn't can only mean that this law was not followed.

I predict that this public-nuisance claim against chain pharmacies will evolve into a claim that pulls the insurance companies (PBMs) into the fight.

When I was trying to plead my case to our county, I skipped, missed, or otherwise overlooked a public nuisance claim against pharmacies. I didn't know that public-nuisance laws existed, but I'm not a lawyer. I was thinking in terms of simple breach of contract between pharmacy and PBM. In this spirit, I was suggesting that Mahoning County try to recover some of the premiums they had been paying to the PBMs that oversaw the prescription drug plan offered to county employees. The specific services PBMs were supposed to administer and the premiums the county had to pay were stipulated in a contract. The county paid so much every month for an employee, and when that employee had a prescription filled at a pharmacy, they paid a deductible. The PBM covered the rest. This was an employee benefit paid for by the employer. Sometimes, these PBMs stipulated which pharmacies the patients could use because those pharmacies had contracts with the PBM. Sometimes, a patient could go to a pharmacy for only the first few fills. After that, they had to use a mail-order pharmacy, which also had a contract with the PBM.

Despite all this complexity, what remains evident are the contracts between the PBMs and the pharmacies, and they all state that "all state and federal laws" must be upheld. Was the contracted pharmacy able to follow all applicable state and federal laws when they dispensed drugs to county employees? A jury was now telling us no, as was the Board of Pharmacy's own survey. If a pharmacy was not abiding by all applicable laws as the contract states, and the PBM promises the county that it would oversee and ensure that they were (also in contract), the county/employer should demand some money back for the premiums it has paid, and perhaps throw in a bit more for the damages caused by the drug misuse.

Think of all the other categories of medications beyond painkillers: diabetic medications, seizure medications, mental health medications, cardiac medications. Pain medications are but one concern. According to federal law, a dangerous drug is a dangerous drug, and death and disease due to poor diabetic compliance or a stroke due to a patient not understanding hypertensive medications are just as serious as opioid abuse. Just because the circumstances surrounding a person's death by stroke or heart attack aren't as obvious as seeing a "foam cone" or meningitis due to an easily traceable vial, the death is certain, nonetheless.

Resisting a system we're all part of isn't comfortable, and it isn't easy. Maybe that's why we see so much lobbying money being dumped into it. A fine dinner with drinks and entertainment that ends with a monetary donation is an easier path to change than cornering a legislator with an uncomfortable truth in the form of a resolution that has been thoughtfully prepared and discussed. The money that purchased a vote may appear to represent the energy needed to solve a problem, but this is where we have been fooled. We cannot be guaranteed an outcome that is in the best interests of the majority if the majority haven't played a role in drafting the solution.

This is a message I brought to college campuses, and although I know they probably only wanted me to show off the cute astronaut suit I climb into to mix drugs, I delivered it whether it seemed comfortable or not.

The purpose of telling my readers these things in this chapter is to suggest that chain pharmacy's problems, our opioid addiction problem, has many actors in many scenes who have all contributed in small ways. Chain pharmacy management is not, and never will be, the only culprit in this story, and yet they are the biggest ones that need to be cut from this story's casting. Even if they are singled out, and billions of dollars in penalties are won from them, support and/or admonishment from other stakeholders in the profession are needed to make the change long-lasting. I mention the depth and scope of the problem to point out the sheer number of players who collectively outnumber everyone except the public itself.

Rarely, if ever, can a single person go up against a culture that involves so many individuals and businesses and expect to move things that are meant for the people to move. One might come close by lighting themselves on fire next to a manifesto they have written, but even then, history tells us that these events are driven by the totality of public discourse. A single speech, lawsuit, or PowerPoint presentation cannot accomplish what an educated and willing public can when they have had enough. And when they have learned enough, and put two and two together, the people will determine all sources of their sufferings and none will escape the change they will bring . . . not chain pharmacies, insurance companies, administrators, educators, county prosecutors, or commissioners. No one was safe when the FDA moved to fix compounding pharmacies, and I suspect this will be the same when agencies are forced by legislation (the people) to move against chain pharmacy.

There was one angle left that I hadn't yet tried, one that the FDA had suggested when I wrote to them. My final period of "irrational exuberance," as Alan Greenspan might call it, arrived after the jury read the result of the public nuisance claim. The Board of Pharmacy was looking at and acting upon the results of their workplace survey, and the people in Lake and Trumbull Counties had spoken. I thought I would take my shot at Uncle Sam, who was the ultimate payor of insurance company-contracted prescription services. If what we were hearing was true, taxpayer money was being wasted, and someone needed to confront the CVSs of the world, who were enjoying $65 billion per year in revenue.

I reached out to the Center for Medicare and Medicaid Services (CMS), the agency within the FDA that oversaw the tax dollars spent on prescription drugs and prescription services. This was, after all, the reason why OBRA-90 was passed in the first place. CMS contracts with prescription insurance companies known as PBMs.

I spent the several days drafting my letter to CMS, which is **Addendum 5.**

Lawyers who work for various counties, townships, or cities might find it of use, should they want to pursue a case against insurance companies. Chain pharmacies are only one piece of this puzzle of deceit; interlocked with them are the insurance companies and mail-order pharmacies they often own, and they are just as culpable as the pharmacies that ultimately dispense the drugs. Taken together, they constitute the entire business model that has driven pharmacist behavior in retail-chain settings, and their pockets are just as deep, if not deeper, than the pharmacies they reluctantly pay for their services.

This is the last piece of correspondence I have written on the subject of chain pharmacy workplace conditions. Should CMS act or another lawyer decide to take up this banner, you can say you heard it here first. Chain pharmacies are being sued now; next up will be the insurance companies that helped drive their activity. I'm the whistleblower. 😃

I emailed a copy of this letter to our EOPA membership list (900 pharmacists) and received only one reply: "Who is approving this stuff."

◆ ◆ ◆

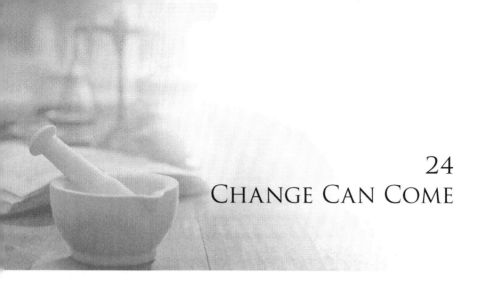

24
CHANGE CAN COME

IN 2022, STATES AND MUNICIPALITIES began to file lawsuits against a major chain pharmacies under the precedent established in the Lake and Trumbull Counties suit, and the amounts being asked for are very large. Now that this cat is finally out of the bag, there will be hundreds, if not thousands, of claims brought against chain pharmacies. It will be up to Walgreens, CVS, Walmart, Rite-Aid, and others to decide if they want to fight one claim after another or bundle their guilt together and agree to one large sum to divide among all claimants.

These types of large class-action settlements are becoming common-place. The price being paid is the total of all the injuries that accumulated over time, plus additional damages to people and property that occurred as a result, and it's reaching into the billions of dollars. Lake and Trumbull counties in Ohio received $650 million; Walgreens was recently ordered to pay a $683 million settlement with the state of Florida; and West Virginia recently settled with CVS and Walmart for $147 million. It's just the beginning, and the stakes are high. At the time of this books printing, and according to The New York Times: "Two of the largest U.S. pharmacy chains, CVS Health and Walgreen Co., announced agreements in principle Wednesday to pay about $5 billion each to settle lawsuits nationwide over the toll of opioids."

The size of the settlements indicate that the offenses were calculated, cut deep, and had all the markings of the moral hazard-type offenses that are difficult for the people to recognize. This is why the offenses went unnoticed for such a long period of time. If these were obvious unlawful acts, someone in the community would have picked up on them. But they weren't. They were of the immoral type that many refuse to see because of the inherent trust "we" have of one another. This trust in mankind, in general, need not be diminished because this once-in-a-generation act committed by many had touched so many. In fact, events such as these underscore our need to be vigilant when protecting the trusting relationships that we enjoy among family, friends, and strangers. Our efforts to maintain a status quo of calm are sometimes just as labor intensive as the efforts we need to put into a good fight when that calm has been shaken.

For nearly a century and a half, the profession of pharmacy has enjoyed a trusting calm about it that in only recent years has been shaken. We pioneered and advanced many drug therapies that have helped to move our country forward in a safe, healthy, and prosperous way. Our pharmacists continue today to help our citizens despite all the financial barriers and corporate challenges placed in their way. And now that the people are coming to our aid, perhaps we might soon see the day educators speak of—when pharmacists are freed from corporate distraction and able to fully utilize the immense wealth of knowledge currently being taught to them. Understanding all that we can do, all that we are willing to do, and our history as chemists and community activists, it would behoove citizens to demand that we use more of our potential for all the good we bring to the table.

Our public cannot and should not allow the immoral acts of one thousand corporate administrators spread out across the country to paint a picture that represents three hundred thousand professionals who had nothing to do with the offenses committed. And those chain pharmacists who found themselves caught in the slave-master relationship that few can ever escape, might now be able to find the professionalism they thought would be theirs when they made the decision to attend a college of pharmacy or university.

Pharmacy can begin a new chapter, and with the help of a vigilant and educated populous, our profession can turn its sights on correcting those areas of our professional lives that only recently have seen failure. First and foremost, chain pharmacists must find a way to gather in the safety of numbers that a professional association affords. They must form an association of their own or inundate those that represent all practice settings and be content with the amount of influence their numbers exert, which could be very large. Either way, they cannot continue to allow assaults on their practice setting to go unchallenged. They must say and do something in a collectively professional fashion, especially when they believe that public safety is at risk. The public can help by asking whether their pharmacist is a member of an organization. Dig just a bit to know if they are on a committee, hold an office, or participate.

Whether or not one might consider another to be more moral or more professional than another because they joined a professional association is a subject for debate in another book. But during these times when we search for morality, professionalism, and good behavior, having such a designation under one's name can go a long way in determining who we want to interact with and who we wish to avoid. Unless your insurance plan prevents you from patronizing a pharmacy of your choosing, exert your influence in ways that are reflective of these types of considerations.

It is possible, and even likely, that you are unable to patronize a pharmacy of your choosing, that you might have to mail away for maintenance medications, or there is no independent pharmacy left near your home. For all the seemingly complex reasons I mentioned earlier that might cause this to be so, changing these dynamics, as large as they might appear to be, are still within our abilities. It is not necessary for someone to understand complicated systems they don't like; it is only necessary to complain when the system is not working as promised. I have offered a basic understanding of how drug dispensing systems work by offering to you the laws under which all are to function. Retail and outpatient pharmacies must operate under the same rules. Only hospital and institutional pharmacies are allowed to follow different rules. Given what you have just read, you now have a foundation from which to recognize illegal and immoral methods of drug dispensing.

Your complaint about a broken or deceptive system can now go further than just a phone call to alert someone that you have different looking pills in your bottle. You have educated yourself on a subject of importance (drugs) and have removed the "information asymmetry" that temps others into taking risks with your health. Now you can hold these complicated systems accountable, and now you can complain intelligently to your boards of pharmacy and legislators. Best of all, you can seek relief from that big and complicated system that has lots of money, either by a letter from your lawyer or from a judge in a courtroom.

I learned just last month that one of the last independent pharmacies in our Youngstown area had closed its doors and sold its prescription files to Rite Aid. I once worked at Campbell Pharmacy years ago when I needed to find extra work, so I was very sad when I heard the news. Few independent pharmacies remain, and those that do struggle to pay their bills. Each one that is lost is to be missed for a myriad of reasons, and as an independent owner myself, it's difficult to begin to explain all the reasons why, so I'll not attempt it here, except to say that things are not going well for the working class.

Over the past several decades, and while we consolidated industries, we have seen employment opportunities—meaningful and honorable jobs for our children–diminish. If we continue down this path, more money will find its way into fewer hands, and Amazon will be the behemoth we asked for. Myself, I'm sad that my father can no longer watch Thursday Night Football because he doesn't subscribe, nor would know how at age 87, to Amazon Prime. Be that as it may, and as my friend Ernie Boyd from OPA often says: "Be careful with what you ask for Christmas because you might just get it."

The public can "break the chains" by patronizing independent pharmacies as much as they can. If your insurance card is accepted there, chances are you will have the same co-pay as you would if you had your prescription filled at a chain pharmacy. Yes, the independent might be a greater distance from your home, they might not have all the neon lights you would see at a chain pharmacy, and their selection of over-the-counter goods might be limited, but exert your influence now that you understand the game that has been rigged against you. These are the small things that we can do in our daily lives that make all the difference in the world.

Check the companies your 401K or pension plan has invested in. Your contributions might help to fund lawsuits and eventual settlements instead of growing a profitable company with good returns. Exert your influence instead of enabling a bad system.

As for myself, my editor informed me that I wrote two books in one, and for clarity's sake I needed to cut. Not wanting to miss an opportunity for a good metaphor, I can say that much of the time I spent trying to fix my profession paralleled my fixing up of old buildings in my town of Lowellville. My highs and lows during the battles I fought for pharmacy brought about my need to escape, and so I retreated to the filth of an old, abandoned building in my hometown. The worse it looked, the more it needed a bulldozer instead of my tools, the more I wanted to bring it back to life.

Our hometown of Lowellville, like many downtowns in the rustbelt, have beautiful and stately buildings crumbling in disrepair because of neglect that comes from the loss of prosperity. Once grand, now only serving as eyesores for our children to see, each sit prominently in our downtown area along the Mahoning River. And just as I would look to the lawful foundation of an association or a practice setting, I would begin in the basement and ensure that the foundation of the building was given attention first. Everything else after that seemed to be gravy once I secured its footing.

I like to work alone and do most of the labor myself. I am on building number eight, and this one is the largest and grandest of them all. It is a three-story brick structure with the façade leaning so far forward that in one year's time it would have collapsed and sealed its doom. The previous owners could not get insurance on it for the safety risks it posed for anyone walking under it. There are times when public danger requires immediate action, and just as with pharmacy, I wanted to act as quickly as possible so the remnants of a grand past would be saved from the insults that threatened it.

I understand that my generation might not be remembered kindly for the way we have treated one another, closed our businesses and manufacturing, and run up debt for our children to pay back. The abundance-to-apathy-to-bondage cycle just happened to land in our time and knowing this makes me want to break the cycle even more. We enjoyed abundant times when I struggled to understand what all the college partying was about, apathetic times when we so few wanted to speak out, and now times of bondage when we feel as though there is nothing we can do to escape our situation. But by educating ourselves in the complexities that bind us, we can work once again and bring prosperity.

The internal anger I felt in my fight to fix pharmacy was calmed each time I stepped back after eleven months of work on a condemned building and was able to see what I had accomplished. My buildings were something I was able to restore. I was able to feel success during a time when pharmacy was delivering nothing but failure, and it's been only within the past year of authoring this book when I realized that the profession was never mine to fix. It's the public who must labor to restore pharmacy to its original condition, and that condition is drafted on paper in the laws that built it.

Those of us who live under its roof are responsible only for maintaining it. The people built retail pharmacy, and they can tear it down if they feel that the foundation on which it is built is beyond repair. Before doing so, understand that OBRA-90 is law and it is where the demolition should stop. Spank the kids who are jumping on the beds and stealing the money from your drawers and remove their allowances. Our house is solid if you are willing to swing your judicial stick and shoo away the rats.

One of the buildings I just finished has a section of brick in the living room that I left exposed. It has two windows with three panes each that faced outside before a room was added years ago. A friend of mine, Brian Komsa, did a reverse glass painting on each of the six panes to depict what in my mind might represent six stages of life, from infancy through adolescence and retirement, and eventually to the final pane representing death. Each depiction is beautifully painted.

With two businesses to run, and another building to fix up, I am not sure when I'll be able to jump from the working-pane to the retirement. I sense, however, that after the completion of this book I will have completed my advocacy for the profession of pharmacy in a record-setting way, with my gutsy lawsuit against my policing agency pushing me over the top. My last pane will come soon enough, but before it does, I want to continue with other interests that are more physical in nature while I am still healthy enough to swing a hammer.

The lessons I learned during my youth, the jobs I left behind, and the mistakes I made contributed to who I would later become as an adult. If repeated insults are numbed by conviction, it's the stuff that change is made of; and with each growing infliction comes our ability to move change to even greater heights. To the one who begins at an early age, it will sometimes seem like "death by a thousand cuts"— be it at the hand of fraternity brothers, colleagues, social media, or district court judges—but it will be the price you pay for the comfort you'll feel in knowing you did the best you could.

I know that sixty will turn into seventy and then hopefully to eighty, when I can reach into my box of home movies and watch them in peace. My hormones and all the cells they stimulate will continue to fade, and I'll reach that last pane of glass in my wall. Should that time come and bring with it the anxiety of knowing I'm about to take my last breath, I hope I'm able to remember enough of my life's accomplishments to calm the feelings of my final goodbye.

THE END

◆ ◆ ◆

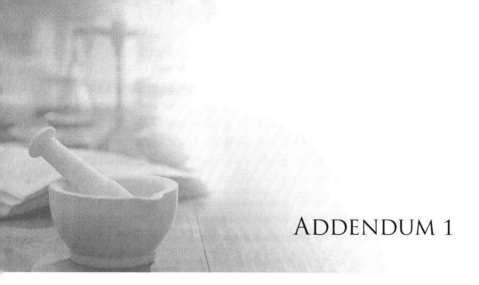

ADDENDUM 1

a. H.R. 5835 (101st): Omnibus Budget Reconciliation Act of 1990 (OBRA-90)

(g) DRUG USE REVIEW-

(1) IN GENERAL-

(A) In order to meet the requirement of section 1903(i) (10)(B), a State shall provide, by not later than January 1, 1993, for a Drug Use Review Program described in paragraph (2) for covered outpatient drugs in order to assure that prescriptions (i) are appropriate, (ii) are medically necessary, and (iii) are not likely to result in adverse medical results. The program shall be designed to educate physicians and pharmacists to identify and reduce the frequency of patterns of fraud, abuse, gross overuse, or inappropriate or medically unnecessary care, among physicians, pharmacists, and patients, or associated with specific drugs or groups of drugs, as well as potential and actual severe adverse reactions to drugs including education on therapeutic appropriateness, overutilization and underutilization, appropriate use of generic products, therapeutic duplication, drug-disease contraindications, drug-drug interactions, incorrect drug dosage or duration of drug treatment, drug-allergy interactions, and clinical abuse/misuse.

(A) PROSPECTIVE DRUG REVIEW.

> (i) *The State plan shall provide for a review of drug therapy before each prescription is filled or delivered to an individual receiving benefits under this title, typically at the point-of-sale or point of distribution. The review shall include screening for potential drug therapy problems due to therapeutic duplication, drug-disease contraindications, drug-drug interactions (including serious interactions with nonprescription or over-the-counter drugs), incorrect drug dosage or duration of drug treatment, drug-allergy interactions, and clinical abuse/misuse.*

> (ii) *As part of the State's prospective drug use review program under this subparagraph applicable State law shall establish standards for counseling of individuals receiving benefits under this title by pharmacists which includes at least the following:*

(I) *The pharmacist must offer to discuss with each individual receiving benefits under this title or caregiver of such individual (in person, whenever practicable, or through access to a telephone service which is toll-free for long-distance calls) who presents a prescription, matters which in the exercise of the pharmacist's professional judgment (consistent with State law respecting the provision of such information), the pharmacist deems significant including the following:*

  (aa) *The name and description of the medication.*

  (bb) *The route, dosage form, dosage, route of administration, and duration of drug therapy*

  (cc) *Special directions and precautions for preparation, administration and use by the patient.*

  (dd) *Common severe side or adverse effects or interactions and therapeutic contraindications that may be encountered, including their avoidance, and the action required if they occur.*

  (ee) *Techniques for self-monitoring drug therapy.*

  (ff) *Proper storage,*

  (gg) *Prescription refill information,*

  (hh) *Action to be taken in the event of a missed dose.*

(11) *A reasonable effort must be made by the pharmacist to obtain, record, and maintain at least the following information regarding individuals receiving benefits under this title:*

  (aa) *Name, address, telephone number, date of birth (or age) and gender.*

(bb) *Individual history where significant, including disease state or states, known allergies and drug reactions, and a comprehensive list of medications and relevant devices.*

(cc) *Pharmacist comments relevant to the individuals drug therapy.*

Nothing in this clause shall be construed as requiring a pharmacist to provide consultation when an individual receiving benefits under this title or caregiver of such individual refuses such consultation.

(3) **STATE DRUG USE REVIEW BOARD.**

(A) *Establishment. Each State shall provide for the establishment of a drug use review board (hereinafter referred to as the 'DUR Board') either directly or through a contract with a private organization.*

(B) *MEMBERSHIP. The membership of the DUR Board shall include health care professionals who have recognized knowledge and expertise in one or more of the following:*

(i) *The clinically appropriate prescribing of covered outpatient drugs.*

(ii) *The clinically appropriate dispensing and monitoring of covered outpatient drugs,*

(iii) *Drug use review, evaluation, and intervention.*

(iv) *Medical quality assurance.*

The membership of the DUR Board shall be made up at least 1/3rd but no more than 51 percent licensed and actively practicing physicians and at least 1/3rd licensed and actively practicing pharmacists.

    (C) **ACTIVITIES.** *The activities of the DUR Board shall include but not be limited to the following:*

        (i) *Retrospective DUR as defined in section (2XB).*

        (ii) *Application of standards as defined in section (2XC).*

        (iii) *Ongoing interventions for physicians and pharmacists, targeted toward therapy problems or individuals identified in the course of retrospective drug use reviews performed under this subsection.*

Intervention programs shall include, in appropriate instances, at least:

    (I) *information dissemination sufficient to ensure the ready availability to physicians and pharmacists in the State of information concerning its duties, powers, and basis for its standards;*

    (II) *written, oral, or electronic reminders containing patient-specific or drug-specific (or both) information and suggested changes in prescribing or dispensing practices, communicated in a manner designed to ensure the privacy of patient related information;*

    (III) *use of face-to-face discussions between health care professionals who are experts in rational drug therapy and selected prescribers and pharmacists who have been targeted for educational intervention, including discussion of optimal prescribing, dispensing, or pharmacy care practices, and follow-up face-to-face discussions; and*

(IV) intensified review or monitoring of selected prescribers or dispensers.

The Board shall re-evaluate interventions after an appropriate period of time to determine if the intervention proved the quality of drug therapy, to evaluate the success of the interventions and make modifications as necessary.

(D) ANNUAL REPORT. Each State shall require the DUR Board to prepare a report on an annual basis.

The State shall submit a report on an annual basis to the Secretary which shall include a description of the activities of the Board, including the nature and scope of the prospective and retrospective drug use review programs, a summary of the interventions used, an assessment of the impact of these ˆ educational interventions on quality of care, and an estimate of the cost savings generated as a result of such program. The Secretary shall utilize such report in evaluating the effectiveness of each State's drug use review program.

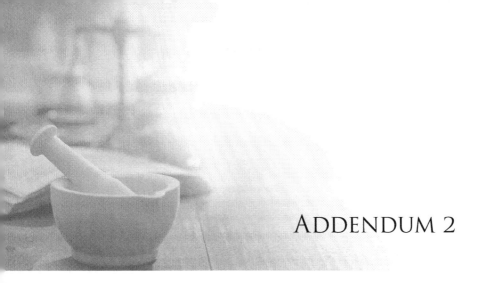

ADDENDUM 2

THE OHIO ADMINISTRATIVE CODE, AS CONTAINED IN OAC 4729-5-21.

Manner of Processing a Prescription, requires the following:

(A) A prescription, to be valid, must be issued for a legitimate medical purpose by an individual prescriber acting in the usual course of his/her professional practice. The responsibility for the proper prescribing is upon the prescriber, but a corresponding responsibility rest with the pharmacist who dispenses the prescription. An order purporting to be a prescription issued not in the usual course of bona fide treatment of a patient is not a prescription and the person knowingly dispensing such a purported prescription, as well as the person issuing it, shall be subject to the penalties of law.

(B) A pharmacist when dispensing a prescription must:

(1) Ensure that patient information is profiled pursuant to Rule 4729-5-18 of the Administrative Code;

(2) Perform prospective drug utilization review pursuant to Rule 4729-5-20 of the Administrative Code.

(3) Ensure that the drug is labeled pursuant to Rule 4729-5-16 of the Administrative Code;

(4) Ensure that a patient is given an offer to counsel pursuant to Rule 4729-5-22 of the Administrative Code.

(5) Ensure that a prescription is filed pursuant to Rule 4729-5-09 of the Administrative Code.

b. OAC 4729-5-18: Patient Profiles

All pharmacies shall maintain a patient profile system which shall provide for immediate retrieval of information regarding those patients who have received prescriptions from that pharmacy.

(A) The dispensing pharmacist shall be responsible for ensuring that a reasonable effort has been made to obtain, document, and maintain at least the following records:

(1) The patient's data record, which should consist of, but is not limited to, the following information:

(a) Full name of the patient for whom the drug is intended;

(b) Residential address and telephone number of the patient;

(c) Patient's date of birth;

(d) Patient's gender;

(e) A list of current patient specific data consisting of at least the following:

(i) Known drug related allergies,

(ii) Previous drug reactions,

(iii) History of or active chronic conditions or disease states,

(iv) Other drugs and nutritional supplements, including nonprescription drugs used on a routine basis, or devices;

(f) The pharmacist's comments relevant to the individual patient's drug therapy, including any other necessary information unique to the specific patient or drug;

c. OAC 4729-5-20: Prospective Drug Utilization Review

(A) Prior to dispensing any prescription, a pharmacist shall review the patient profile for the purpose of identifying:

(1) Over-utilization or under-utilization;

(2) Therapeutic duplication;

(3) Drug-disease state contraindications;

(4) Drug-drug interactions;

(5) Incorrect drug dosage;

(6) Drug-allergy interactions;

(7) Abuse/misuse;

(8) Inappropriate duration of drug treatment; and

(9) Food-nutritional supplements-drug interactions.

(B) Upon identifying any issue listed in paragraph (A) of this Rule, a pharmacist, using professional judgment, shall take appropriate steps to avoid or resolve the potential problem. These steps may include requesting and reviewing an Ohio Automated RX Reporting System report or another state's report, pursuant to paragraph (D) of this Rule, and/or consulting with the prescriber and/or counseling the patient.

(C) A prescription, to be valid, must be issued for a legitimate medical purpose by an individual prescriber acting in the usual course of his/her professional practice. The responsibility for the proper prescribing is upon the prescriber, but a corresponding responsibility rest with the pharmacist who dispenses the prescription. Based upon information obtained during a prospective drug utilization review, a pharmacist shall use professional judgment when making a determination about the legitimacy of a prescription. A pharmacist is not required to dispense a prescription of doubtful, questionable, or suspicious origin.

d. OAC 4729-5-22: Patient Counseling

(A) A pharmacist or the pharmacist's designee shall personally offer to provide the service of counseling pursuant to paragraph (B) of this rule to the patient or caregiver whenever any prescription, new or refill, is dispensed. A pharmacist shall not be required to counsel a patient or caregiver when the patient or caregiver refuses the offer of counseling or does not respond to the written offer to counsel. If the patient or caregiver is not physically present, the offer to counsel shall be made by telephone or in writing on a separate document accompanying the prescription or incorporated as part of documentation, in a conspicuous manner that is included with the prescription. A written offer to counsel shall include the hours a pharmacist is available and a telephone number where a pharmacist may be reached. The telephone service must be available at no cost to the pharmacy's primary patient population.

(B) In the event a patient or caregiver accepts an offer to counsel or requests counseling, a pharmacist, or an intern under the personal supervision of a pharmacist, shall counsel the patient or caregiver. Such counseling may include, but is not limited to, the following:

(1) The name and description of the drug;

(2) The dosage form, dose, strength, frequency, route of administration, and duration of drug therapy;

(3) The intended use of the drug and the expected action;

(4) Special directions and precautions for preparation, administration, and use by the patient;

(5) Common adverse effects or interactions and therapeutic contraindications that may occur, including possible methods to avoid them, and the action required if they occur;

(6) Techniques for self-monitoring drug therapy;

(7) Proper storage and disposal;

(8) Prescription refill information;

(9) Action to be taken in the event of a missed dose, and

(10) The pharmacist's comments relevant to the individual's drug therapy, including other necessary information unique to the specific patient or drug.

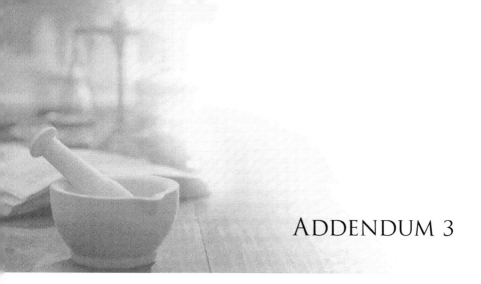

Addendum 3

An Original mailing sent to chain pharmacists
in 1996

NATIONAL ASSOCIATION
of
EMPLOYEE PHARMACISTS

the Voice of the Employee/Chain Pharmacist   Volume 1, Number 1   1996

CAN THE MAJORITY AFFORD TO REMAIN SILENT?

The current state of pharmacy might lead one to believe that someone's interests are not being protected. The PEW REPORT estimates a surplus of 40,000 pharmacists by the year 2000 and has recommended reducing the number of pharmacy schools by 25% by the year 2005. The public is mandating actions to serve us with notice of their discontent at the high cost of medication misuse. Our professional environment grows busier and more confusing in the wake of higher volume, lower margins, and 3rd Party management. Even more sad is the report that we have the second highest risk of suicide among more than 230 occupations analyzed by NIOSH.

We are a concerned group of Employee/Chain pharmacists asking for you to give heartfelt consideration to what we believe is an important pharmacy issue. We are the National Association of Employee Pharmacists (NAEP), and we believe that a professional organization to directly represent the interests of pharmacy's largest practice setting is long overdue.

OH NO! NOT ANOTHER ASSOCIATION!

We have national associations that represent Hospital, Independent, Clinical, Consulting, and Scientific pharmacists. We also have associations that represent pharmacy educators, pharmacy lawyers, pharmacy boards, pharmaceutical manufacturers, pharmaceutical distributors, owners of pharmacy chains, managed care pharmacy, and many more. Those who benefit from joining their own practice setting association can likewise join the professional organizations available to all. The 50 state associations represent all pharmacists within given boundaries and APhA represents all pharmacists within the 50 states. So, how has it come to pass that in the midst of so many organizations representing so many interests that the Employee, who constitutes the majority, has been without such benefits?

NAEP IS ABOUT DEMOCRACY PROTECTING THE MAJORITY!

The right of a particular practice setting to elect their own officers, establish committees, attend conventions, and receive publications that exchange ideas and information is not reserved for Hos-

pital, Independent, Consulting, or the myriad of other interests within the profession. Pharmacy democracy is for all practice settings to use in order to share experiences, reach consensus, send representatives, receive grants, inform its members, and find solutions to problems. Can this or any other profession afford to have such a silent majority? Has our lack of involvement given consent to resolution of pharmacy issues that may not have been in the best interests of the majority, and therefore possibly the profession as a whole?

Pharmacy has long claimed that it has lacked unity and strength. The forces outside of pharmacy have shown both, and as a result have greatly impacted the profession. The potential threats are as real as our inabilities to position ourselves as providers of managed care if we choose not to become involved. Those who have called for the unification of

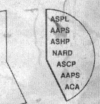

existing organizations have overlooked the 65% of the profession in the best

ASPL
AAPS
ASHP
NARD
ASCP
AAPS
ACA

NAEP

position to give pharmacy what it lacks.

The profession needs to look at the Employee Pharmacist as the untapped potential from which to gain strength and unity. A vast array of trusted professionals from which to draw input, ideas, and involvement has long been overlooked. NAEP is about giving equal representation and support to individual Employee Pharmacists who care enough about the profession and its future to join with other professional pharmacy groups in determining how best to protect it.

cont. on pg. 2

NAEP Protects the Majority *cont. from pg. 1*

NAEP is Growing to Fill a Tremendous Void

Our membership now reaches into several states. We are the young and working many busy hours and we are the retired reflecting back and seeing how much the profession has changed. Those who have joined NAEP feel we can do for ourselves what others have been attempting to do. Pharmacy can no longer afford such a silent majority giving consent for others to decide what is best when they have only a survey or opinion poll on which to assess the full impact. A fully informed representative to JCPP, the APhA House of Delegates, or to speak before ACPE who is deciding the issue of the Pharm.D. on behalf of an absent Employee consensus is the top priority of NAEP. We are beginning by reaching the 110,000 Employee Pharmacists to inform them of this professional imbalance and NAEP's determination to correct it.

The November 6, 1995 cover of "DRUG TOPICS" (THE TRAGIC TRUTH) says more about our need to become more active than any words we could write in this mailing. It speaks volumes of our responsibility to ourselves. The PEW REPORT tells of our responsibility to the profession while the multibillion dollar cost of medication misuse reminds us of our duty to the public. We invite you to join NAEP so that together we can actively participate with other practice setting associations to set a course that is best for all of pharmacy.

Raymond R. Carlson, R.Ph.
NAEP - Ohio

Associations by Settings

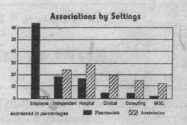

expressed in percentages ■ Pharmacists ▨ Association

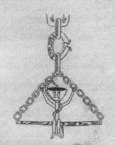

A SAMPLING OF SENTIMENT

" I am an Employee Pharmacist and I feel that an association of this type is greatly needed. I want to thank you for your work in this area." (K.R., MICHIGAN)

"Please send me any information you can along with any suggestions on what I can do to help." (W.J., PENNSYLVANIA)

"I have been on every side of retail pharmacy ... there is a need for a voice of the Employee... add my name. (D.H., VERMONT)

"I just got home from another 12 hour shift. I will visit some of my pharmacy friends who will want to know more about NAEP. (M.M., FLORIDA)

"I am very interested in the association ... tell me how I can help. (H.N., ILLINOIS)

"I think there are a large number of pharmacists not presently involved in pharmacy groups due to the lack of promotion or interest in the Employee Pharmacist." (C.B., CALIFORNIA)

"There is much we can accomplish and much we need to accomplish." (D.B., OHIO)

" *Those who deny freedom to others deserve it not for themselves and under a just God can not long retain it.*"
Abraham Lincoln

Article of the third ...... *Congress shall make no law respecting an establishment of religion, or prohibiting the free exercise thereof; or abridging the freedom of speech, or of the press, or of the people peaceably to assemble, and to petition the government for a redress of grievances.*

Our constitution was written to protect and promote the well-being of our nation. It allows those with common interests and common knowledge to decide what is best for themselves and the public. Our freedom of speech allows us to address the microphone, our freedom of press allows us to receive entertaining and informative publications, and our right to peaceful assembly allows us to attend conventions and meetings to share new ideas and experiences. Our unwillingness to make use of these rights that many have died to protect makes us unable to redress any governing body. Is it possible that the largest practice setting of our nation's most trusted profession is without grievances? Are we without ideas to share with other organized segments of pharmacy that will better our ability to serve the public? These rights have been secured for us to better care for ourselves and the public. If we fail to care for ourselves, the public will not allow us to care for them.

Their Freedoms Are Our Freedoms As Well!

American Association of Pharmaceutical Scientists
American Association of Colleges of Pharmacy
American Chemical Society
American College of Apothecaries
American College of Clinical Pharmacy
American Society of Consultant Pharmacists
American Society of Health System Pharmacists
American Society for Pharmacy Law
Drug Information Association
Health Industry Manufactures Association
Health Insurance Association of America
National Association of Boards of Pharmacy
National Association of Chain Drug Stores
National Association of Managed Care Pharmacy
National Association of Medical Equipment Suppliers
National Association of Parenteral and Enteral Nutrition
National Association of Retail Druggists
National Association of Wholesaler-Distributors
National Pharmaceutical Association
National Wholesale Druggists Association
Nonprescription Drug Manufacturers Association
Parenteral Drug Association
Pharmaceutical Manufacturers Association
Private Label Manufacturers Association

Ricky from Anytown, U.S.A. says:
I've got it!
Why not join
our own association?
The kind
everyone else
seems to have.
We would elect
our own officers,
form committees,
discuss problems & ways to solve them
... and then
we would send a representative
to voice our own opinion and cast our own vote!

IMPORTANT UPDATE:

NAEP WASTES NO TIME TO REPRESENT YOU:

The American Pharmaceutical Association invited Ray Carlson, R.Ph. (NAEP-Ohio) to discuss Employee quality of worklife and professional representation issues at the August 24th APhA-APPM Executive Committee and Section Chairs meeting in Washington D.C. A motion was passed to establish a task force to assess Employee Worklife conditions, seek standardization of 3rd Party Plans, and recommend name and/or structure changes to APhA Sections to provide for better representation.

APhA is our association to protect all of pharmacy. As NAEP is to one setting, so too is APhA to all. We have opened the door enough to see that together we must turn the tide for our setting and the profession. NAEP will have a seat on this task force and we will need and welcome your input and ideas. *Please, make the time to respond!*

NAEP GOALS AND OBJECTIVES

- To improve public health
- To advance the efficiency of Employee Pharmacy
- To promote the utilization of professional skills within the practice of Employee Pharmacy
- To advance the standing of its members and the practice of Employee Pharmacy
- To serve as a forum for debate on issues pertinent to the practice of Employee Pharmacy
- To promote the awareness of current legislation and to stimulate legislation favorable to these objectives
- To unite the practice of Employee Pharmacy for the purpose of these objectives

NO SEAT, NO VOTE FOR THE MAJORITY

MEMBERS OF THE JOINT COMMISSION OF PHARMACY PRACTITIONERS (JCPP)	MEMBERS OF THE APHA HOUSE OF DELEGATES
• American Association of Colleges of Pharmacy	• American Association of Colleges of Pharmacy
• American College of Apothecaries	• American Association of Pharmaceutical Scientists
• American College of Clinical Pharmacy	• American College of Apothecaries
• American Pharmaceutical Association	• American College of Clinical Pharmacy
• American Society of Consultant Pharmacists	• American Institute of the History of Pharmacy
• American Society of Health System Pharmacists	• American Society of Consultant Pharmacists
• American Association of Retail Druggists	• American Society of Health System Pharmacists
• National Council of State Association Executives	• National Pharmaceutical Association

ACCORDING TO THE LATEST:

...Employee Pharmacists represent over 60% of the profession.

...Less than 40% of pharmacy enjoys the benefits of more than 20 national associations while the remaining single majority has not had one ... *until NAEP.*

...Pharmacists are 3½ times more likely to commit suicide than the general public.

...Growing use of technicians will trim between 14,000 and 45,000 FTEs from the demand for R.Ph. services. Automation, Robotics, and Centralization will cut 19,000 to 60,000 FTEs.

...There is a National Association of Pharmacy Technicians.

...Eight Independent Drug Stores close daily.

...K-Mart Corp. closed 75 pharmacy departments on July 31st. The closings were traced to underperformance in a cutthroat prescription drug marketplace. (256 Pharmacists affected)

...The U.S. NEWS and WORLD REPORT August 26th cover story is entitled "DANGER AT THE DRUGSTORE" ... an investigative report worth considering.

...NARD's High Noon II is scheduled for September 16-20, 1996.

...110,000/194,570 pharmacists representing one practice setting is without a voting seat on JCPP.

...For every dollar spent on medication use ... an equal dollar is spent to correct medication misuse.

...TIMETABLE FOR THE PHARM.D. January 1996 - January 1997: (Second comment period): Hearings on proposed changes and submission of written comments to occur at various professional organization meetings. **A professionally organized consensus [not a survey] on behalf of Employee Pharmacy (60%), regardless of position, failed to meet the first comment deadline.**

...The National Association of Chain Drug Stores (NACDS) has 135 active drug chain members. Members minimum annual dues: $2640.00.

...Employee Pharmacists fill 75% of the more than 2 billion prescriptions filled annually in the U.S.

...Target Stores has introduced a fully automated pharmacy system at its store in Edwina, Minn.

We Have Heard All the Reasons Why Not:	NAEP Offers Some Reasons Why:
• Employe Pharmacists are professionally apathetic.	• Employe Pharmacists are highly trained caring professionals who constitute the majority of our nations most trusted professionals.
• Management takes care of the employee.	• Certain responsibilities of the profession are best not delegated.
• NACDS represents the employee.	• NACDS is a trade association of chain executives and pharmacy suppliers.
• There are so many other associations.	• Only the Employee/Chain Pharmacist as a specific practice setting has been without representation.
• No complaints: Good salaries & many jobs available.	• Low margins, High volume, Robotics, Increased use of techs, Centralization. Surpluses are predicted and surpluses bring down wages.
• What are you going to do for me?	• Find out how you feel about the mandatory Pharm.D., Tech certification, High Volume, Break Periods, 3rd Party, Closed Networks, Etc. Then vote Yea or Nay **ON YOUR BEHALF.**
	• Inform and educate you ... and give you the means to inform others.

Use This NAEP Application for Membership

NATIONAL ASSOCIATION of EMPLOYEE PHARMACISTS
MEMBERSHIP APPLICATION FORM

FOR YOUR OPINION, CONSENSUS, AND VOTE
TO PROTECT, INFORM, AND REPRESENT

NAEP is a Professional Association of Employee/Chain Pharmacists

ACTIVE MEMBERSHIP DUES: $65.00 ANNUAL
Please make your check payable to:
N A E P
P.O. Box 83, Lowellville, Ohio 44436

NAME _____   WORK _____

ADDRESS _____   ADDRESS _____

CITY _____ STATE _____ ZIP _____   CITY _____ STATE _____ ZIP _____

PREFERRED MAILING ADDRESS: ☐ HOME   ☐ WORK

LICENSURE: _____
STATE   LICENSE #   YEARS LICENSED   OTHER STATES LICENSED

EDUCATION: _____
SCHOOL   DEGREE(S) HELD

TELEPHONE: HOME ( ) _____   WORK ( ) _____

FAX: ( ) _____   E-MAIL ADDRESS _____

The NAEP Newsletter contains editorial comments in addition to current statistical information concerning issues of concern for Employee Pharmacists.

We welcome your letters and comments, and hope you will share your opinions with us.

HELP NAEP TO SERVE YOU:
CHECK ALL THAT APPLY.

____ AVG. 0-24 HOURS PER WEEK

____ AVG. 25-39 HOURS PER WEEK

____ AVG. 40 OR MORE HOURS PER WEEK

____ WORK MORE THAN 1 LOCATION (FLOATER)

____ BEEN WITH COMPANY OVER 5 YEARS

____ FILL 100 SCRIPTS A DAY

____ FILL 100-200 SCRIPTS A DAY

____ FILL OVER 200 SCRIPTS A DAY

PRIORITIZE THESE ISSUES
NUMBER FROM 1 THRU 5
WITH #1 BEING THE HIGHEST

____ INSURANCE CONFUSION/LACK OF STANDARD FORMATS

____ MANDATORY PHARM.D.

____ PHARMACIST BREAK PERIOD

____ HIGH VOLUME

____ INABILITY TO PRACTICE AS EDUCATED

TELL US WHAT YOU THINK

_____

_____

_____

_____

_____

_____

_____

_____

_____

_____

_____

_____

_____

_____

_____

_____

_____

_____

Use back side of sheet if needed.

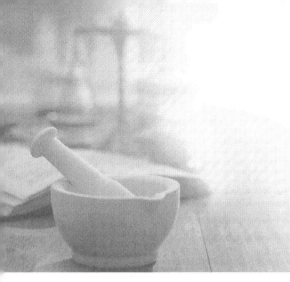

Addendum 4

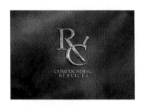

Raymond R. Carlson, R.Ph.
RC Compounding Services, LLC
RC Outsourcing, LLC

Toni L. Bisconti, Ph.D., Michael T. Vale, MA, & Jennifer Sublett
University of Akron

OBRA-90: Pharmacy Compliance with Counseling and Profiling in Ohio Residents

*As part of the current study, we surveyed approximately 600
Ohio adult residents who have had at least one interaction with
a pharmacy over the past year. Specifically, we examined whether
the general adult public is interested and/or offered medication
counseling by their pharmacists. Additionally, we sought to gauge*

compliance with respect to pharmacists' ability to obtain patient-specific information prior to filling a prescription. We explored general attitudes about pharmacies/pharmacists and other issues and/or interactions that occur at the pharmacy.

Information collected during the Fall of 2018 is housed anonymously on the survey system Qualtrics through the University of Akron. Before any surveys were distributed, UA's Institutional Review Board reviewed and approved the study. After that process, we used a word-of-mouth and crowd surfing method in order to collect data via listserves and social media. All the researchers involved in the project are from the NE Ohio area, so the counties in which the information was collected was clustered in that area (although 39 of the 88 Ohio counties had at least one participant).

According to Federal (OBRA-90) and/or Ohio Board of Pharmacy Rules (OAC 4729), a pharmacy must offer the service of medication counseling on all matters that fall under the pharmacist's professional judgement with each individual to whom a prescription is being dispensed. That medication information should include but is not limited to the following:

- *The name and description of the medication*
- *The dosage form, dosage, route of administration, and duration of the drug therapy*
- *Any special directions and precautions for preparation, administration, and use of the drug*
- *Common severe or adverse side effects and/or drug interactions*
- *Techniques for self-monitoring drug therapy*
- *Proper storage*
- *Refill information*
- *Action to be taken if I miss a dose*

According to Federal Law (OBRA-90) and/or Ohio Board of Pharmacy Rules (OAC 4729), the dispensing pharmacist shall be responsible for ensuring that a reasonable effort has been made to obtain, document, and maintain at least the following records:

* *Full name of the patient for whom the drug is intended*
* *Residential address and telephone number of the patient*
* *Patient's date of birth*
* *Patient's gender*
* *Known drug-related allergies*
* *Previous drug reactions*
* *History of our active chronic conditions or disease states*
* *Other drugs and nutritional supplements including OTC drugs used on a routine basis*
* *Use of medical devices*

The primary goal of the project which Mr. Carlson spearheaded was to examine whether pharmacists are complying with this law. Because of his own vested interest in the information, Mr. Carlson used a University of Akron research team to create and distribute the survey. Broadly speaking, according to approximately 600 consumers in Ohio, pharmacists are NOT complying with the offer to counsel law and are falling short of what would be considered a "reasonable attempt" to obtain patient-specific information for profiling purposes. Please see the data below for specific questions and answers.

If you have specific questions about the methodology or data collection, please contact the Transitions, Resilience and Identity— Lab (uatrilab@gmail.com or Dr. Toni L. Bisconti (tb33@uakron.

edu). If you have any questions about the content or the substance of the information, contact Mr. Ray Carlson (rccompounding@ sbcglobal.net).

DESCRIPTIVE DATA REPORT

N = 627 Ohio residents (Answers to questions ranged from 541–627 due to missing data)

Age
N = 623
Range: 18–84; *M* = 45.37

Gender
N = 626
Female = 495; 79%; Male 126; 20%; Transgender = 5; .08%

County
N = 626

Allen .8%	Franklin 2.7%	Mahoning 22.6%	Seneca .3%
Ashtabula 1.4%	Geauga 1.0%	Medina .6%	Stark 1.0%
Butler .2%	Greene .2%	Meigs .2%	Summit 33.9%
Carroll .3%	Hamilton .5%	Montgomery .6%	Trumbull 1.0%
Columbiana .8%	Huron .2%	Ottawa .3%	Van Wert .2%
Crawford .2%	Lake 21.7%	Pickaway .2%	Vinton .2%
Cuyahoga 4.1%	Licking .3%	Portage 1.6%	Warren .5%
Delaware .5%	Logan .2%	Richland .2%	Wayne .2%
Erie .2%	Lorain .6%	Ross .2%	Wyandot .2%
Fairfield 2.7%	Lucas .2%	Scioto .2%	

***78.2% of the sample came from 3 counties; all of which are in NE Ohio

Do you pay out of pocket for your prescriptions or do you use a prescription insurance card?

    N = 627
    12.4%   paid out of pocket
    87 .6%   **paid through insurance card**

On average, how many times a month do you regularly have a prescription dispensed in your name?

    N = 627
    18.2%   fill 0 prescriptions
    66.5%   fill 1–3 prescriptions
    2.2%   fill 7–10 prescriptions
    1.6%   fill 10+ prescriptions

Where do you fill your prescriptions?

    N = 627
    7.2 %   Independently owned
    26.6%   Big Box
    53.3%   Stand alone retail
    9.1%   Mail Order
    4.3%   Hospital Pharmacy

SECTION 1: COUNSELING

It is clear when interacting with the pharmacy staff which person(s) is the actual pharmacist.

59.6%	Yes
40.4%	No

Your regular pharmacist knows your name.

23.3%	Yes
76.7%	**No**

At the time a script is dispensed to you, how much time do you *typically* spend talking with your pharmacist (NOT solely the staff) in regards to it?

70%	**None (70%)**
19.5%	**Less than a minute**
9.6%	2–5 minutes
1%	5–10 minutes
0%	Over 10 minutes

How often does the pharmacist discuss the following topics with you when you pick up your scripts?

a. Name and description of the medication

50.8%	Never
23.4%	**Rarely**
15.3%	Sometimes
5%	Often
5.5%	Always

b. The dosage form, dosage amount, route of administration and duration of the drug therapy

53.3%	Never
23.2%	Rarely
13.8%	Sometimes
4.4%	Often
3.4%	Always

c. Any special directions and precautions for preparation administration and use of the drug

46.7%	Never
23.2%	Rarely
19.5%	Sometimes
5.5%	Often
5%	Always

d. Common severe or adverse side effects and/or drug interactions

61.3%	Never
19%	Rarely
12.6%	Sometimes
4.5%	Often
2.5%	Always

e. Techniques for self-monitoring drug therapy

77.6%	Never
13.8%	Rarely
5.5%	Sometimes

2.5%   Often

1.5%   Always

f. Proper storage

73.1%   **Never**

13.4%   **Rarely**

9.6%   Sometimes

2.4%   Often

1.5%   Always

g. Refill information

63.4%   **Never**

19.3%   **Rarely**

11.6%   Sometimes

3.7%   Often

2%   Always

h. Action to be taken if I miss a dose

76.8%   **Never**

14.6%   **Rarely**

6.4%   Sometimes

1.3%   Often

.8%   Always

How frequently has your pharmacist made an error (not related to price or insurance) when dispensing your script?

78.2%	Never
16.95	Rarely
4.7%	Sometimes
.2%	Often
0%	Always

Do you believe this error would have been caught with more direct conversation with your pharmacist at the time you ordered or received your script?

63.1%	Yes
36.9%	No

SECTION 2: THE OFFER TO PROVIDE MEDICATION COUNSELING SERVICES

When I have a question about my medication *at* the pharmacy, I feel like the pharmacist is too busy to bother.

32%	Never
21.3%	Rarely
26.1%	Sometimes
12.5%	Often
8.1%	Always

When I have a question about the medication I have received from a mail order pharmacy, I feel as though there are too many barriers to call and talk with a pharmacist.

19.2%   Never
14.1%   Rarely
23.9%   Sometimes
16.9%   Often
25.8%   Always

Are you required to sign anything when you pick up your scripts?

84.3%   **Yes**
15.7%   No

Has it been made clear to you what it is you are signing when you pick up your script?

58.8%   **Yes**
41.2%   No

SECTION 3: THE LAW

According to Federal and State law, a pharmacy *must offer the service of medication counseling* on all matters that fall under the pharmacist's professional judgement with each individual to whom a prescription is being dispensed. That medication information should include but is not limited to the following:

* The name and description of the medication
* The dosage form, dosage, route of administration, and duration of the drug therapy

* Any special directions and precautions for preparation, administration and use of the drug
* Common severe or adverse side effects and/or drug interactions
* Techniques for self-monitoring drug therapy
* Proper storage
* Refill information
* Action to be taken if I miss a dose

Prior to reading the above definition, did you know that there is an "offer to counsel" law?

38.4%	Yes
61.6%	No

According to Federal and State law, a qualified pharmacy staff member must *offer to provide medication counseling* to the customer whenever any prescription is dispensed.

How well do you think the above offer to provide medication counseling is being made to you?

19.5%	Not at all
24.5%	Not very
28.4%	Somewhat
18.4%	Very
9.3%	Extremely

Are you aware that you were declining the service of medication counseling when you signed at the time you received your medication?

38.8%	Yes
61.2%	No

How necessary do you think this law is?

(Missing data 86/627, 13.7%)

.7%	Not at all (.7%)
4.1%	Not very (4.1%)
26.6%	Somewhat (26.6%)
42.7%	**Very (42.7%)**
25.9%	Extremely (25.9%)

How often do you think *your* pharmacist(s) complies with this law?

5.2%	Never
25.9%	Rarely
28.6%	Sometimes
18.1%	Often
22.2%	Always

Given that a medication counseling session could take 5–10 minutes per drug, how often do you think that *your* pharmacist(s) could reasonably comply with this law?

5.2%	Never
5.7%	Rarely
9.6%	Sometimes
13%	Often
66.5%	**Always**

According to Ohio drug dispensing law, the dispensing pharmacist is responsible for making sure that a reasonable attempt has been made to obtain the following information prior to processing your prescription. Please rate how often this information is asked of you:

Your full name

5.2%	Never
5.7%	Rarely
9.6%	Sometimes
13%	Often
66.5%	**Always**

Your address and telephone number

24.8%	**Never**
21.1%	**Rarely**
15.5%	Sometimes
11.3%	Often
27.3%	Always

Your date of birth

4.4%	Never
4.1%	Rarely
6.4%	Sometimes
9.6%	Often
75.4%	**Always**

Your gender

76.6%	**Never (76.6%)**
9.1%	Rarely (9.1%)
3.6%	Sometimes (3.6%)
2%	Often (2.0%)
8.7%	Always (8.7%)

Drug related allergies you have

40.4%	**Never**
20.3%	**Rarely**
15.7%	Sometimes
7.8%	Often
15.8%	Always

Previous reactions to drugs you have had

78.2%	**Never**
16.9%	**Rarely**
4.7%	Sometimes
.2%	Often
0%	Always

History of or active chronic conditions or disease states

67.4%	**Never**
14.5%	**Rarely**
9.1%	Sometimes
3.9%	Often
5%	Always

Other prescription drugs you are taking

55.9%	**Never (55.9%)**
16.1%	Rarely (16.1%)
16.1%	Sometimes (16.1%)
4.5%	Often (4.5%)
7.5%	Always (7.5%)

Nutritional supplements you are taking

77%	**Never**
11.9%	Rarely

5.7%   Sometimes

1.6%   Often

3.7%   Always

Nonprescription drugs you are taking

76.6%   **Never**

12.3%   Rarely

5.2%   Sometimes

2.7%   Often

3.2%   Always

Mean (1.43)

Any medical devices you use (c-pap, catheter, insulin pump, nebulizer, etc.)

80.7%   **Never**

10.7%   Rarely

3.2%   Sometimes

1.4%   Often

3.9%   Always

Given that a Federal law enacted in 1990 established rules of information gathering and counseling and was meant to *"thwart the abuse and misuse of prescription drugs,"* how important a role do you feel that pharmacists should play in the control of drug distribution?

3.7%   Not at all

5.5%   Not very

23%   Somewhat

32.6%   **Very**

35.1%   **Extremely**

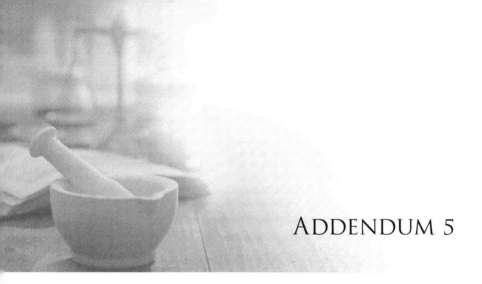

EASTERN OHIO PHARMACISTS ASSOCIATION
Ashtabula, Columbiana, Geauga, Lake, Mahoning, Trumbull
102 East Water Street, Lowellville, Ohio 44436

January 24, 2022
Chiquita Brooks-LaSure
Department of Health and Human Services
Centers for Medicare & Medicaid Services
7500 Security Boulevard
Baltimore, MD 21244-1850

Dear Chiquita,

Given the recent headlines regarding the state of retail pharmacy throughout the U.S., the Eastern Ohio Pharmacists Association would like to express our concerns regarding nationwide compliance with H.R. 5835; Drug Use Review; otherwise known as OBRA-90. Our concerns for patient safety were shared with the

FDA who in turn suggested we contact CMS since it is your agency that provides funding and apparent oversight of monies spent.

Various state pharmacy boards, NABP, APhA, and others have issued statements in response to pharmacist complaints about stressful workplace conditions as well as consumer complaints involving errors. Our nation's misuse and abuse of drugs, both opioid and non-opioid, is no secret.

In Ohio, the citizens residing in two of the counties our association represents recently won a jury trial claiming chain pharmacies created a "public nuisance" (Lake and Trumbull Vs. CVS, Walgreens, Walmart). Giant Eagle and Rite Aid settled out of court. Likewise, our Ohio Board of Pharmacy's survey on workplace conditions (April 2021), containing many hundreds of chain pharmacist complaints, points to retail chain pharmacies operating business models in ways that create unsafe drug dispensing conditions. We have confidence that these conditions exist in most all states.

CMS is funding drug dispensing which is too fast and as such is in essence potentially unlawful. As CMS now actively considers the purchasing arrangements involving pharmacies, Pharmacy Benefit Managers (PBMs), and other 3rd party non-dispensing contracted entities, we ask that you first reread and consider the public intentions contained in H.R. 5835. These entities no matter their complexity, have no authority to establish business models through muddied contracts which act or otherwise influence lawful dispensing duties in such ways that risk public health, strain public funds, or stress pharmacy dispensers who are charged with upholding the law.

OBRA-90 and various Boards of Pharmacy rules are clear as to what the public expects from pharmacies and the PBMs who contract services on their behalf. In exchange for receiving federal tax dollars, states were to promulgate rules and establish a Drug Use Review Board. Reference to these dispensing expectations is clear in both HHS and CMS guidance.

One would believe that after nearly 30 yrs. of OBRA-90 compliance and perhaps hundreds of billions of dollars spent, the public would be drug and disease savvy, free from the criminal intent of abusers, and enjoying a marketplace of affordable drugs. But that is not where we find ourselves today:

* *More than 100,000 overdose deaths in the U.S. in 2021.*
* *More than 50% of patients are non-adherent with medications at any time.*
* *Some 20% of hospital admissions are due to misuse of prescription drugs.*
* *State pharmacy Boards expressing concerns about unsafe workplace conditions.*
* *Chain pharmacists and technicians voicing concerns about the unsustainable and unsafe workload throughout the U.S.*
* *A successful Public Nuisance Claim made against chain pharmacies for their role in the spread of opioid pills in Trumbull and Lake Counties in Ohio.*
* *Ridiculously priced prescription drugs, including now over-inflated generics drugs.*
* *Countless losses of life and property are associated with all classes of prescription drugs.*

OBRA-90 establishes the grounds on which payments are to be made and so we request you audit the essential categories outlined in the Act: Gathering of Patient Information, Thoughtful Drug

Utilization Review, Patient Profiling of Relevant Information and Pharmacists' Comments, and Patient-Pharmacist Counseling. One study by the University of Akron suggests less than 10% compliance in all major categories, less than 5% are counseled in any meaningful way with over 90% claiming less than 2 min. total spent talking to a pharmacist. Only 30% believe their pharmacist would know their name.

We see that CMS recognizes the complexity and unsustainability of our current drug reimbursement system and is taking action to rein it in. However, in CMS-4192-P there is no mention of compliance with respect to outcome measures linked to OBRA-90 and no apparent efforts planned to enforce it. It is troubling that any action taken to correct funding would be void of conversation about the people's expectations as laid out in H.R. 5835. We believe there need to be genuine compliance considerations to this law which the people have already placed before us and before additional layers of bureaucracy addressing other 3ʳᵈ party areas of concern are implemented.

Compliance oversight when funding OBRA-90 participants will protect the public from the dangers of services rendered when they themselves are not the payor and as such feel less inclined to protect their own consumer rights. As financial transactions are left to third parties (PBMs), so too is the responsibility to safeguard the people from those who would take advantage of them. We believe it is the ultimate responsibility of CMS to provide these public safeguards in exchange for payments.

The Eastern Ohio Pharmacists Association is appreciative of CMS' efforts to address what has been a long-waged war against lawful drug dispensing in the U.S. We ask that you recognize pharmacists as a critical cog in a rapidly spinning wheel and address the misleading role of corporate pharmacies, mail-order pharmacies, and PBMs with whom they are contracted and perhaps even own. At their current pace, are these entities able to dispense drugs according to CMS contracts which state that "all State and Federal laws are to be followed when rendering prescription services"?

CMS should look at the number of prescriptions dispensed over time. No pharmacist can safely dispense the numbers we suspect for as long as we suspect. The laws governing dispensing make no mention of an automated system replacing the professional judgment of the dispensing pharmacist. In reading the Act, corporates' assumption that a system on autopilot could possibly be the public's intent, or an alternative, is at best a far stretch.

OBRA-90 required each state to create a Drug Use Review Board. While we cannot speak to the effectiveness of other state review boards, Ohio's, unfortunately, meets quarterly for an average of 55 minutes. There is little mention in meeting minutes of growing concern for the use (amount/duration) of opioids.

Other states receiving federal funds must have missed these trends for the length of time it took for us to recognize the number of citizens who became addicted. Misinterpreted data was coupled with dispensing systems that did not allow for human interaction, profiling of information, or simple one-on-one counseling to ferret out abuse. When the math began to add up, patients were met with across-the-board reductions of doses allowed. Minimizing the issue to a "numbers problem," not a recognized human problem which failed to determine legitimate pain from non-legitimate, brought about new rules which drove patients to purchase street vendor doses of unknown content to replace those which were once trusted and "lawfully" dispensed. This was a dispensing system failure, not a board or committee failure. OBRA-90 mandates a review of each prescription upon dispensing.

A law enacted in 1990 calling for Drug Use Review should not have marked the beginning of a period when seeds of addiction were planted. This law was meant to prevent such happenings. We cannot now know the full extent of costs associated with the misuse of all categories of prescription drugs. Just to clarify, opioids are but one of many dangerous drugs covered by OBRA-90.

Inquiries of these sorts will lead one to determine whether a prescription drug was dispensed according to the reasonable wishes of the people or hurried out of a cue. No contract, industry-accepted or not, has the authority to undermine dispensing laws. Revisiting CMS's contracts do show, on its face, intentions to comply. Contracts sometimes specifically mention OBRA-90 as well applicable state law.

Corporate pharmacies have the advantage of enjoying relationships with plan sponsors, PBMs, and mail-order pharmacies. Opaque relationships, opaque payments, and "take it or leave it" contracts have decimated independent pharmacies and the human interactions that the people sought to secure in 1990. These advantages occur by skirting the rules and agencies must now find a way to recognize the deviance despite the opaque nature of the players. At this moment, evidence abounds that unjust and ill-gotten volumes threaten public safety, create unlevel playing fields, limit shared labor of important responsibilities, and deepen the waste of financial resources.

It seems difficult to imagine that a system wrought with lawsuits, medication errors, pharmacist burn-out, and safety inquiries is such a system—a contracted system—which could warrant inflated and opaque payments, many of which never reach the actual dispenser, and for which the people continue to make. The public should expect compensation back and cessation of payments to such a system if it has been determined by CMS, who is the ultimate payer, that payment for mandated dispensing services meant to keep the public safe are being made under potentially breachful pretense. The public should not expect their leaders to drift further from laws they have already enacted because of the size of the problem acknowledged, the number of stakeholders involved in its growth, or the slow creep of our own moral hazards.

PBMs are contracted with pharmacies, and both parties receive payments from CMS for services rendered. These services must be assured to be of lawful intent and in keeping with what a trusting public expects but know little about. Lawful adherence in a meaningful way also protects the profession of pharmacy so that we, the pharmacists, are released from hastened business models that work to undermine the people's protection under OBRA-90. Drawn from your payments for drug dispensing services are the 3rd party slices of a pie which have removed valuable assets and cherished time from the very front-line pharmacists who are the defined dispensers. Most importantly is the understanding that these responsibilities are to be satisfied before the drug is dispensed before commissions are called and data reviewed and before societal problems are born. Pharmacy and its lawful dispensing activity are the pie, and a meaningful slice must remain for payment to recognize its importance to public safety.

Pharmacists are highly educated professionals and are charged with an "equal and corresponding responsibility with physicians" to ensure that prescription drugs are for legitimate medical purposes. The public has seen these lawful duties removed from the pharmacists' control and they acknowledge our hurried state in what they see happening when having a prescription filled. Pharmacists are simply unable to properly dispense prescription drugs in the times allowed. It is not possible to read OBRA-90 and envision a business model that could comply within a 60-second timeframe. A hurried pharmacist is unable to attach valuable knowledge and oversight to drug dispensing when time constraints, corporate metrics, vaccinations, and 3ʳᵈ party billing issues dominate their workplace conditions.

None of these concerns should be misconstrued as anti-competition or a failure to recognize economies of scale where the people benefit from cost reductions. However, rules exist to level the playing field and create safe expectations for consumers. Just as one would be concerned for the quality of bread if a baker today were selling each loaf for a penny, one should be extremely concerned when the article of commerce in question is a dangerous drug being dispensed by a licensed pharmacist at a loss.

Our trusted agencies receive data, read headlines, speak to colleagues, and make payments. This larger picture painted should entice agencies to look for areas where we might have strayed. OBRA-90 and the subsequent rules promulgated by pharmacy boards is that big picture and it has been our profession's 800 lb. gorilla for many prosperous yet debt-ridden years.

This law expects pharmacists to be able to assume control and take the necessary time prior to dispensing, without exhaustion and amidst comfortable levels of professional human interaction, to ensure those who take prescription drugs understand the importance of adherence, exchange additional information with the pharmacist who then makes entries into patient profiles, and lastly, that the inherent dangers of the drugs which they are about to consume are worth more than the payments assigned by 3ʳᵈ parties (non-dispensers). Despite all 3ʳᵈ party shortchanging, and with irony, they ultimately return to take the value back (claw backs), striking again at the missed fine print detailing OBRA-90.

We believe the essential elements of OBRA-90 is where agency gap analysis should begin. Any payment made to those who have contracted to provide drug dispensing services to some 27 million Medicare and Medicaid patients need to be made on the verified assumption that H.R. 5835 is adhered to.

We understand the desire to conveniently use Covid as the scapegoat for the stresses we now confront. EOPA, however, passed a Resolution in March of 2018 asking our Board of Pharmacy to investigate compliance with dispensing laws/rules. It was a concern being raised in many other states. Covid only showed our frailty and further unveiled our raped system of prescription drug dispensing and laws meant to have allowed for certain levels of professional cushion.

Public expectations contained in this Act are too high for us to ignore chaotic workplace conditions, sustained dispensing volumes, or hesitant complaints from licensed pharmacists. What has been interpreted by many, even those within our own profession, as the mundane chore of dispensing, is in fact the essence of the clinical and caring activity sought by the people when they enacted OBRA-90. Unfortunately, it now reads like an eerie premonition if we strayed.

No amount of data collection, committee review, or cubical pharmacy activity can replace the inherent safety contained in this Act. A renewed focus on the people's law will slow the process and create accountability; it will make information gathering more meaningful, hold entities to the lawful essence of contracts, limit *grey areas to exploit, inform the public about drugs and disease management, and provide beneficial outcomes for the dollars spent.*

If we fail to make the changes necessary, both in funding and compliance oversight, the public will when they are educated as to what it really means to legally dispense a federal legend drug. They never expected protection from drug misuse by licensed pharmacists count by five when they enacted H.R. 5835. Nor did they expect automated care, or that they would receive $1.00 worth of dispensing service because a PBM claimed that to be its value. Certainly, they never expected to endure the drug use issues they now face or the incredible amounts they would pay to underwrite its cost. Maybe they did?

Thank you for your consideration. We hope to hear a reply and pray to see action in this area of pharmacy dispensing law compliance. Still, we will continue with our efforts, and thank you for your time.

Respectfully,

RAYMOND R. CARLSON, R.Ph.

President—EOPA

Founder—Pharmacists Have Patients

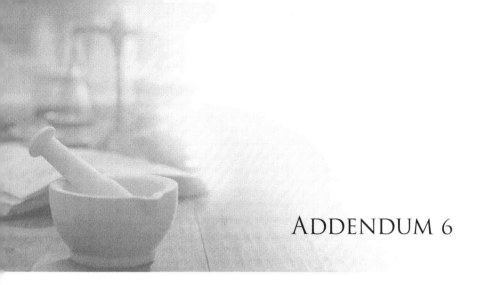

ADDENDUM 6

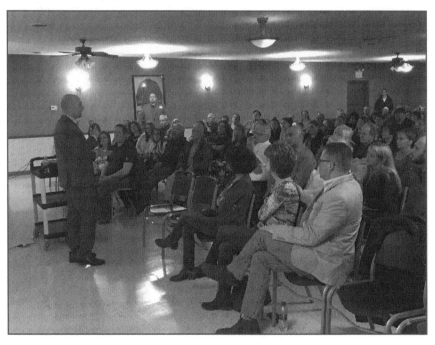

Senator Joe Schiavoni speaks at the RC Public Forum

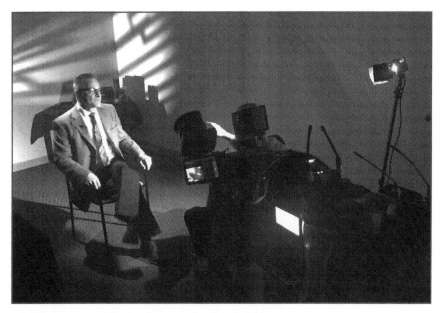

Ray interviews with TV-5 News, Cleveland, Ohio

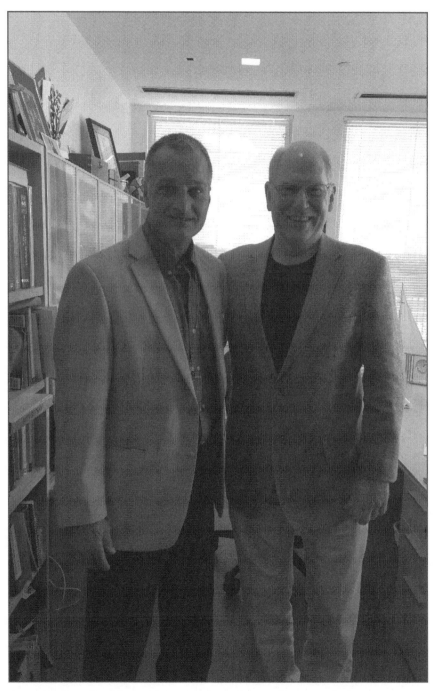

Ray with Tom Menighan, CEO, American Pharmacists Association

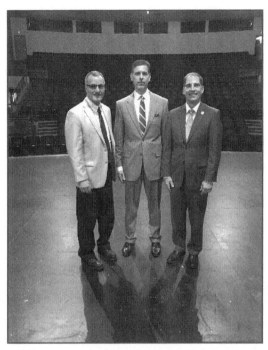

Ray with B. Douglas Hoey, CEO of the National Community Pharmacists Association, and Steve Martin, dean of ONU's Raabe College of Pharmacy.

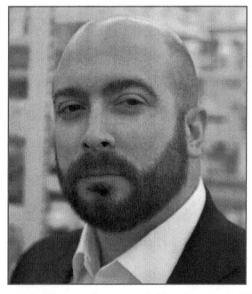

Antonio Ciaccia, Ohio Pharmacists Association Director of Government and Public Affairs and CEO of 46brooklyn Research.

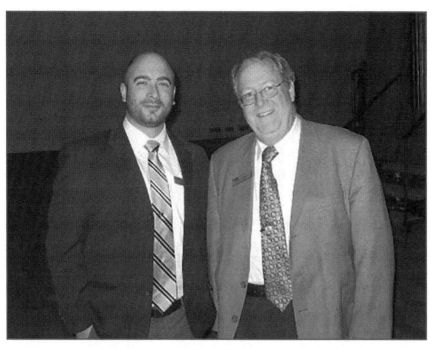

Antonio Ciaccia with Ernie Boyd, retired executive director of the Ohio Pharmacists Association

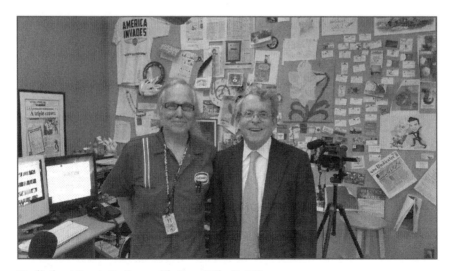

Radio host Louie B. Free with Gov. Mike DeWine

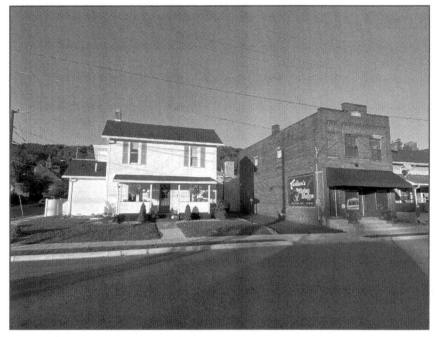

Building #5 and #6 restored in downtown Lowellville, Ohio

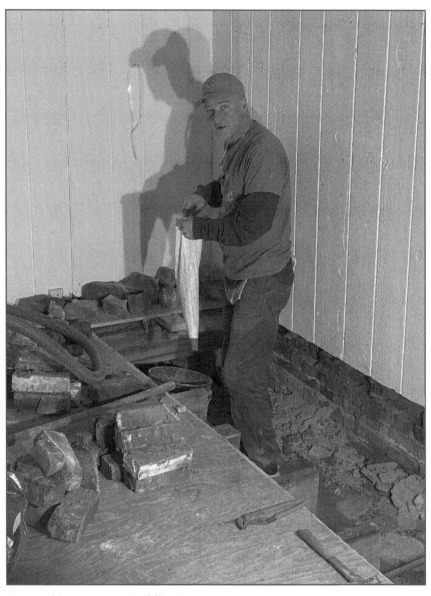

Ray working to restore Building #7

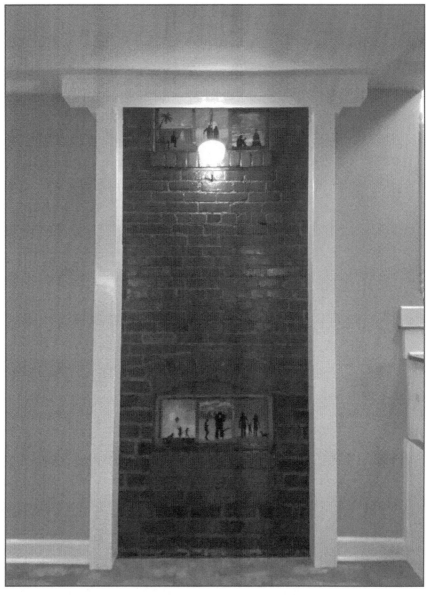

Reverse painting of six stages of life by artist Brian Komsa

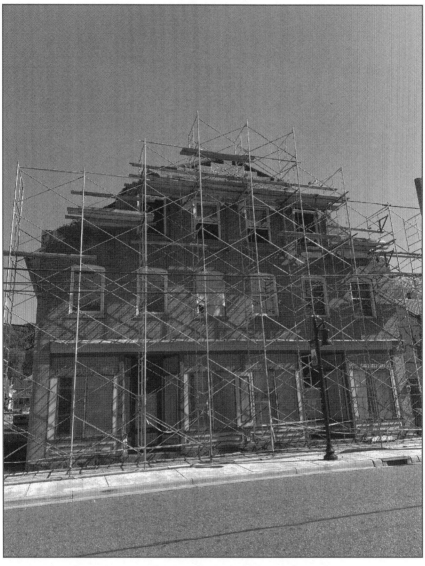

Restoration begins on Building #8 in downtown Lowellville, Ohio

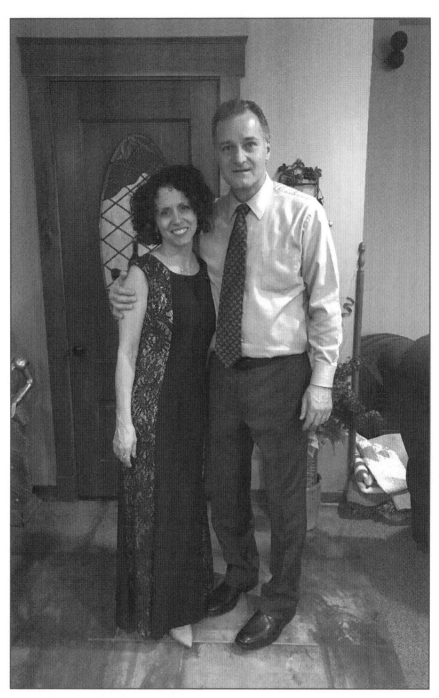

Ray and Lori Carlson

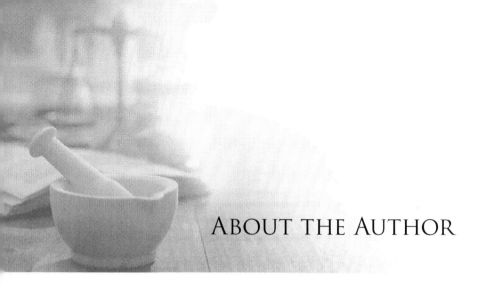

ABOUT THE AUTHOR

RAY CARLSON is the owner of RC Outsourcing, an FDA-licensed 503B Outsourcing Facility in Lowellville, Ohio. He graduated from Ohio Northern University's Raabe College of Pharmacy in 1985. Over his long career, he has worked at independent, chain, hospital, and home infusion pharmacies. Ray is a past president of the Ohio Pharmacists Association and Eastern Ohio Pharmacists Association and a former PCAB Surveyor. He is currently a member of APhA, OPA, EOPA, and the owner of a 503A pharmacy, RC Compounding Services, in Poland, Ohio, where he works with his wife, Lori, and daughter Emily. He has another daughter, Sarah, a nurse, and a son, Ray, Jr., an electrician.

Made in the USA
Monee, IL
20 January 2023

25767595R00201